STAY SLIM WHILE
YOU QUIT SMOKING

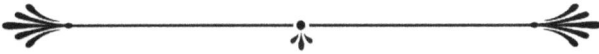

Theodore W. Robinson

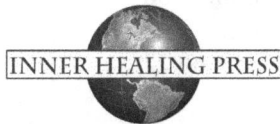

INNER HEALING PRESS

Stay Slim While
You Quit Smoking

ISBN 0978654137

An Inner Healing Press Publication
www.innerhealingpress.com
www.centerforinnerhealing.com

ACKNOWLEDGMENTS

There are so many people to thank, it's hard to know where to start. Well, not really. First, most importantly, a full acknowledgment and thank you to Theresa Rodriguez, who has been with me for almost a decade as a loyal assistant and paralegal. Theresa has been a source of inspiration and information about everything in my life. Without her, this book would never have been written or completed. There are no words that can express how grateful I am for her friendship, loyalty and limitless creativity, knowledge, patience and wisdom. And, of course, for Jillian, her new daughter who brightens my world every day.

I also give thanks to my teachers - Leonard Jacobson, Walter Belling, Tom Carpenter and Gary Craig. Each has offered insightful information and/or techniques about another part of the puzzle we call life. Each has affected how I view life and what I share with others. I thank each of them individually from the bottom of my heart.

I also give thanks and have great gratitude for all those students who have offered insights through their questions and comments. They have profoundly changed what I share with others and how I view the world and hopefully how those who read this will change as a result.

Finally, I thank God for the inspiration to write this book in the hope that it will help change the landscape of our nation and perhaps the world by helping people finally end their life-threatening habit of smoking and over-eating.

TABLE OF CONTENTS

INTRODUCTION

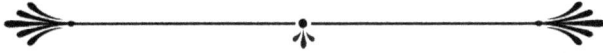

The primary concern for most people who are thinking about kicking the smoking habit is whether they will be successful or not. However, another key concern most smokers express is whether they are going to gain weight after they stop smoking. Most think they will gain weight. While this could be just another rationalization to justify not quitting, a number of people do gain weight when they quit smoking. In other words, many often trade a smoking habit for an eating habit.

The good news is you <u>don't</u> have to gain weight when you stop smoking. That's what this book is all about. However, it will take some attention and conscious awareness to avoid putting on extra pounds as you quit a life long habit that many have used as an appetite suppressant in the past.

This book will help you gain that awareness and give you plenty of practical advice on how to quit smoking and stay slim while you do it. It will also give you ways to control your eating habits and help you improve your overall lifestyle at the same time.

If that sounds like a good goal and something you'd like to accomplish, then read on. This is the beginning of a new way of life for you as a Non-Smoker - for Life.

CHAPTER 1

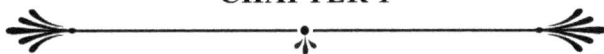

YOU <u>CAN</u> STAY SLIM AND QUIT AT THE SAME TIME

It's a generally accurate perception that when people stop smoking, many of them gain weight. Yet, it doesn't have to be that way. For years, perhaps decades, you've been clogging up your taste buds with tar and other harmful chemicals which caused them to become less effective. That's one of the reasons why food doesn't hold the same interest for smokers as it did before they started smoking - if they can even remember back that far.

First, when you finally quit smoking, the cells in your taste buds start to naturally cleanse themselves and start to regenerate. That's when you start to taste your food again and it will often taste a <u>lot</u> better. Your natural instinct to eat more food will often kick in because you're enjoying your food more and eating can often get out of control if you don't pay attention. In fact, if you aren't conscious of what you're doing, you can quickly put weight on and once it's on, it's a lot harder to take off than to keep it off in the first place. We're going to give you a lot of information on how to become more aware and keep the weight off before it gets a head start on you and your body.

Smoking naturally suppresses your appetite. The effect of the chemicals in tobacco smoke cut down your appetite and reduce your interest in eating. Whenever you smoked in the past, you automatically kept your weight down by suppressing your appetite. Once you stop smoking and the chemicals are no longer entering your system, that suppressed appetite no longer has anything holding it back - and at the same time everything starts to taste better . . . before you know it . . . well, you get the picture.

On top of that, many people use a cigarette in order to fulfill their need to have something in their hand or mouth to quiet their nerves or lessen their anxiety. When they stop smoking, that urge often continues but there's no cigarette to hold in their hand. They often replace the cigarette with food. Before they know it, they're putting on weight again. Is the picture getting clearer?

Obviously, it's very important to eliminate the propensity to overeat after you quit smoking. A recent study done at Johns Hopkins University concluded that quitting smoking can contribute to the onset of Type 2 Adult Diabetes. Ironically, it's not because smokers stop smoking but because stopping often leads to obesity and obesity indirectly leads to diabetes. The study concluded that it was best to stop smoking and also do something about not putting weight on as a result of quitting. That's the very purpose of this book.

When you consider all three of the forces that coalesce and contribute to form a single urge, it can become very powerful and it's not surprising that people put weight on easily - especially when they're not consciously thinking about it.

However, it doesn't <u>have</u> to be that way. You don't necessarily have to put on weight when you stop smoking. Instead, quitting smoking can actually become an incentive to bring greater consciousness into your life so you can live with more awareness and mindfulness about every aspect of your life. That will ultimately bring a better lifestyle for you in many ways, keeping you slim and eventually bringing more peace, harmony and happiness into your life. In effect, once you quit smoking, you can live a better life.

So how do you do all this? What's the answer? By becoming more conscious of how you feel, what you're thinking, what you're eating and by being more aware of what you're doing whenever you put food into your mouth, you'll be able to control your weight better and stay slim fairly easily.

It's the unconscious eating habits of people that get them into trouble. The hand-to-mouth habit that has no bearing on hunger or need, but is simply a way of satisfying some other emotional need that remains unfulfilled or becomes more pronounced once you stop smoking. In fact, it's the unconscious thoughts, feelings, unbridled emotions and our judgements of them that make most of us dissatisfied and unhappy in the first place. When we bring more consciousness into our lives we usually find we are far more happy, peaceful and fulfilled. This book will help you do exactly that and help you remain slim while you quit smoking - for life.

BACK TO THE BEGINNING

Before we go any further, let's take a step back to smoking itself and discuss the best ways to quit. This is for all those reading this book who are still contemplating quitting smoking and haven't yet taken the steps to finally stop or for those who may have quit a number of times for varying periods and always went back to it.

The good news is that hypnosis has finally been acknowledged as the best and most effective means for quitting smoking. Research shows that when hypnosis is used correctly, the success rate is above 66%. When compared to the success rates of trying to quit on your own (5%), using behavioral therapy (25%) or using Nicotine gum, the patch, or prescription drugs, etc. (25%), **hypnosis is the most effective means of quitting smoking**. In fact, there is no other method supported by research that even comes close.

While 66% sounds impressive, it still means that 1/3 of those smokers who use hypnosis alone will still likely go back to smoking. That's not acceptable to us. That's why we added another healing component, Emotional Freedom Technique to hypnosis and made it the most comprehensive package of techniques available today. As a result, your likelihood of success will increase substantially to the 90 percentile range.

There are a number of reasons for this, but the primary one is that smoking is nothing more than a habit. Habits are based upon beliefs that have become established in the subconscious mind and subsequently become the programming for your actions.

For example, the way you relate to the world is a reflection of your beliefs which are based upon all your prior experiences. Your actions and reactions are a response to those experiences. In fact, it's those actions and reactions that often become so ingrained in you that they become your unconscious habits. Smoking is a perfect example of an unconscious habit. Take a look at your own behaviors around smoking. If you look closely, you'll notice your actions are not well thought out or mindful, but instead are usually just repeated actions to quell anxiety or any number of other urges or negative emotions.

For example, if you feel that every time you start a personal relationship, you end up being victimized and hurt, you'll probably start to avoid starting new relationships. It's a reasonable and rational conclusion to make that if you avoid getting into relationships in the first place, you can't get hurt or feel victimized. Simple avoidance can then become a way of life for you and this can then lead you to become habituated to it.

The problem is, by avoiding relationships, you also remain alone and alienated from the world and unhappiness becomes a way of life too. That's not a great approach to life and relationships, yet it is how our subconscious mind tends to deal with hurt and rejection.

With cigarettes, most people start out smoking as adolescents who just wanted to be part of the "in-crowd" or be cool. However, over the years, after that particular scene moved on and there was no more "in-crowd" to join, smoking just remained as a habit. That habit usually adds other emotional triggers to it such as becoming an antidote to tension, stress or anxiety or is used as a finish to a meal or intimacy. After awhile, smoking simply becomes a bad habit and becomes so ingrained that it seems impossible to change the habit.

In fact, while most smokers have tried and failed to quit repeatedly, the truth is, their subconscious minds just never quite made the shift that was needed in their inner belief system. As a result, it was inevitable that they "couldn't quit" in their outer perspective if their inner programming never changed beforehand.

As author Glenn Poveremo says: "If you want to change your life, you must first change your mind."

As we mentioned earlier, hypnosis has been proven to be the most effective means of quitting. The reason is simple. Once a person is hypnotized, the Hypnotist helps them directly change their belief system within the subconscious mind through direct suggestions and other insights. Hypnosis bypasses the critical factor of the conscious mind. The critical factor of the conscious mind stands like the "Sentinel at the Gates" of the subconscious mind. It only lets in thoughts that are already consistent with the beliefs the subconscious mind already embraces.

That's how the subconscious mind works. Once you've made up your mind about something, you are more prone to hang onto it than to change it. For example, if you're a member of a certain political party from a very early age, no amount of arguing or logic is going to change your mind. Your mind has embraced a certain belief system and nothing is going to change it - because of the critical factor of the conscious mind which is intended to maintain your existing belief system intact. We call this a built-in resistance to change within the mind.

Again, the critical factor of the conscious mind evaluates any new thought that is introduced to you and it will be "stopped at the gates" until the conscious mind is sure it's consistent with the subconscious mind's existing belief system. If the new thought is consistent with your prior thoughts, conclusions and beliefs, then it will be allowed to pass into the subconscious mind, which is innocent by nature and prone to accept whatever is introduced to it.

On the other hand, if a new thought is **inconsistent** with the existing thoughts and beliefs of the subconscious mind, then the critical factor of the conscious mind will stop it cold and reject it. It will often attach what it deems a "rational" reason for it's rejection, like it might harm you or hurt you or it might conclude that it doesn't make any sense. In fact, the conscious mind will rationalize its choice by bringing in any other "facts" it feels it needs to justify its rejection. It will reject it no matter what facts are offered because it's inconsistent with its previously existing belief system. No matter how hard you try to introduce those new thoughts or beliefs and go through all the motions to show you've accepted them, the same result will occur. They will be rejected. That's the job of the critical factor of the conscious mind and it's just doing its job.

USING HYPNOSIS TO QUIT SMOKING

With hypnosis, the Hypnotist assists the person to enter into a hypnotic trance (which is actually very focused attention), effectively setting the conscious mind aside so it no longer acts as the "Sentinel at the gates." The Hypnotist will then give direct suggestions to the subconscious mind consistent with the new behavior or understanding that is desired. Most people misunderstand this concept and think they're going to be "put to sleep" because Hypnotists often say "sleep" to assist the person to enter into a trance.

Another misconception is that most people believe they won't hear what's going on or understand anything while they're in hypnosis. That's not the case at all. When you're hypnotized, you hear everything that's going on and you can actually sense your conscious mind evaluating everything as it is said by the Hypnotist. In such situations, the conscious mind simply doesn't choose to interfere with what is being said to the subconscious mind while it is deeply absorbing everything being said. At least not usually. If something untoward or inappropriate is said by the Hypnotist, your innate protective mechanisms will kick in and you'll come out of trance and interrupt what's being said. But that rarely happens.

Once the Hypnotist is speaking directly to you while you're in a state of hypnosis, they give you different suggestions regarding quitting your smoking habit. That can be done with direct suggestions that you will no longer smoke or a number of other ways such as demonstrating why smoking is so bad for you. The specifics are unimportant, however, by doing this the Hypnotist is effectively helping you change your mind and its belief system about smoking at the subconscious level. Once the new thoughts are given to you, the Hypnotist will then offer you additional mental suggestions to reinforce the original suggestions so they will be carried out by you in your everyday life and be reinforced by common things you see or do in your life.

After the first session, it is usually beneficial to have at least one reinforcement session just to make certain that the suggestions have been fully accepted by the subconscious and are incorporated into your daily life. It's also important to make sure your inner mind hasn't done anything to undermine the suggestions after leaving the office.

Perhaps the most important aspect of quitting smoking is your mental attitude. If you say to yourself, "Gee, I hope this works" or, "I'll give this technique a try," the process is unlikely to work for you. Your mind is already set up for failure as soon as you use either of those two words "Hope or Try."

On the other hand, if you say to yourself, "I like those ideas - I know they're going to work," that's when the suggestions are fully accepted into the subconscious mind and they do work. This is a very important distinction. If you choose to fully embrace the suggestions you receive with full acceptance and with a mind set that they are going to work - they are far more prone to working than with any other mind set.

Remember, the purpose of making these suggestions is two-fold. One is to establish direct changes in your belief system. The second is to change your habit from being self-destructive to a healthy one. Any habit can be changed in 21 days. The primary goal is to change your destructive habit into a healthy one and maintain it for at least the first 21 days. When you do that and keep it going for the first three weeks, you'll be well on your way to permanently eliminating smoking from your life - for life.

The same advice holds true when it comes to unconsciously eating food. If you suddenly realize you've overeaten the day after you've binged on junk food, you're a prime candidate to use hypnosis to change that behavior. In the same way hypnosis can help you overcome smoking, it can help you overcome overeating. The same type of subliminal suggestions about food are made to you while you are in a trance and before you know it, your eating habits will change for the better and you will become more mindful of what you eat - when you eat.

USING EMOTIONAL FREEDOM TECHNIQUE
TO KEEP THE WEIGHT OFF

Another important part of the package we've developed is to teach those who want to stop smoking Emotional Freedom Technique or EFT. This is because, despite changing your basic belief system at its very roots in the subconscious mind, there are often other negative emotional aspects that still drive or trigger your bad habits or adverse behavior such as smoking and overeating. It could be the need to have something in your hands or mouth all the time (*i.e.*, an oral fixation) or anxiety that needs to be satisfied in an attempt to feel normal. These are usually unconscious or subconscious behaviors that go unnoticed on a conscious level. They often drive you to do things you'd rather not do, but usually don't notice that you're doing them until it's already too late.

The best way to address these unconscious behaviors including harmful smoking and overeating habits is to bring consciousness to them. However, for those who can't seem to do that on their own, then the best thing you can do is learn Emotional Freedom Technique. EFT will directly help you stop smoking and overeating in conjunction with hypnosis and will also eliminate the underlying emotional issues and energy imbalances that drove you to smoke and/or to overeat in the first place. You do this by recognizing when you're feeling driven to do things that you don't really want to do, but do them anyway.

The best part of learning EFT and using it to help you cement your choice to quit smoking is that it increases your odds of quitting to almost 100% effectiveness. Even though hypnosis will help you change your underlying belief system, sometimes an old urge to smoke may arise in certain situations and if you don't know how to handle it on the spot, you may succumb to it and smoke again. With EFT and the DVDs that we've designed, you can literally stop any urge to smoke in its tracks! Once that happens and the urge passes without you picking up a cigarette, the road is clear for your continued success as a non-smoker for life!

To learn EFT, just go to the Emotional Freedom Technique chapter. If you would rather see exactly how it is done, you may visit our web site at hypno-eft.com and then go to the EFT page. There is a video tutorial you can follow as well as an illustrated manual and a handy EFT on a Page and a diagram you can print and keep as a guide.

With EFT, all you need to do to change your smoking or eating habits is verbally acknowledge your bad habits as they arise and then tap on the various meridian access points until those negative thoughts go away. For example, if you have a big urge to eat some cake - or even a whole cake - all you have to do is say words to the effect of, "Even though I really <u>want</u> to eat that cake, I love and accept myself nonetheless," or say something as simple as, "I really <u>want</u> that cake. I wish I could have that cake right now." You then say portions of those phrases as you tap each of the meridian access points, such as "I want that cake" or "I have to have that cake right now."

You may be thinking "Why would I say I <u>want</u> the cake, when my real reason for using the technique is to stop me from eating it?" Well, it's because EFT is the only <u>negatively stated</u> technique and it works best that way. That's because of the underlying premise of EFT which is: "All negative thoughts, negative behaviors, self-limiting beliefs and pain come from a blockage in the meridian system." In other words, when your meridians are blocked, your normal life force energy (known as "chi") can't flow and that's when negative thoughts and beliefs arise.

We use negative words when describing these habits in order to "bring up" and fully feel the negative emotions attached to them. That way, we actually <u>increase</u> the blockages in the meridians at the same time. We do this because when the meridians are more fully blocked, we then have more to tap away and we get better overall results for our clients.

When we do EFT, we tap with the first two fingers of the dominant hand (index and middle fingers) at each meridian access point in order to unblock the meridian attached to it. It's similar to tapping the top of a straw that has a little fluid - like milk - left in the middle of it. The tapping dislodges the blockage and the life force energy can flow again through the meridians. As a result, the negative emotions are resolved quickly and effectively.

If using EFT on your own doesn't fully satisfy your needs and you still remain firmly entrenched in overeating or smoking, then you may want to visit a local EFT practitioner and delve into the emotional issues that may be driving your behavior when you know they don't serve you any longer. Your EFT practitioner will assist you in accessing and eliminating those negative urges in short order so you'll be able to control them if they ever arise again. This will bring greater consciousness to your eating habits which will then allow you to be more in control of your life and more at peace.

After you've learned EFT, then it's time to use the following wording suggestions to support the change you've already started in your smoking habit. These are specific Set-Up phrases that will help you address many of the basic things that drive over-eating. You may adopt or use any of them or you may modify any of the suggestions to fit your personal needs. Always remember that the wordings are intended to <u>bring up your negative emotions to their fullest extent</u>. The purpose of this is to establish the blockages in your meridians. Again, we do this because when the blockages are fully in place, we use EFT to tap them away and we get better results than if we try to tap away an emotion that is not being felt at the time. Remember, with EFT you have to "feel it to heal it."

Once you are experiencing the negative feelings, you know that the meridians are blocked. At that time, you simply tap on the access point of each meridian with two fingers to unblock the meridians and allow the normal life force energy to flow again. That allows the meridians to balance themselves out naturally and the negative emotions or self-limiting beliefs will disappear quickly and you'll be left with neutral or positive emotions or feelings. The negative drives will also naturally disappear in the same fashion.

Here are the Set-Up phrases you may wish to use. (Remember, once you finish the Set-Up, you then tap on all the meridian access points and say "reminder phrases" which are just part of the Set-Up phrases. You can simply take a few words from the Set-Up and use them as reminders as you go along to each point. Follow the example.):

Set-Up:

"Even though I know once I quit smoking I'm going to want to eat more, I love and accept myself fully and completely." (Say this 3 times as you tap on the Karate Chop point)

Sequence:

Eyebrow Point - EB - "I'm afraid I'm going to overeat."
Side of Eye - SE - "I really want to eat more now."
Under Eye - UE - "I can't control my eating."
Under Nose - UN - "I'm afraid I'm going to get fat."
Collarbone - CB - "I just know I'm going to fail at this."
Under arm - UA - "This is never going to work for me."
Top of Head - TH - "Why is everything so difficult?"

Secondary Set-Up:

"Even though I'm already feeling a little better, I still don't believe this is going to work for me. I'll never be able to control my eating while I'm doing my best to not smoke. Yet, I love and accept myself no matter how this all turns out."

Sequence:

EB - "I'm actually feeling a little better already."
SE - "I still don't trust any of this."
UE - "I feel stupid doing all this tapping stuff."

UN - "I wonder if it will really work for me?"
UM - "I actually am feeling a little tingling sensation."
CB - "I like this and think its really going to work for me."
UA - "I am actually feeling better already."
TH - "I like this already. I know it will work for me."

Additional Set-Ups:

"Even though I know I won't be able to control my eating habits once I quit smoking and I'm going to get fat, I love and accept myself anyway."

"All of my friends have gotten fat when they quit smoking and I'm really worried that's going to happen to me too. Yet, I love and accept myself nonetheless because I know I must stop smoking, no matter what else happens to me."

"Once I stop smoking, I'm afraid it's going to take all my will power just to remain smoke free. How am I ever going to watch what I eat at the same time? I'm really worried I'm going to get fat, yet I love and accept myself fully and completely nonetheless."

"Now that I've stopped smoking, why shouldn't I allow myself some other excesses, like food, to reward myself for quitting smoking? So what if I put on some weight. Yet, I know this is all my mind rationalizing my behavior and I don't really want to gain weight, but I'm really afraid I won't be able to control myself any longer. And I love myself nonetheless and accept myself fully and completely."

"Why does everyone expect so much from me? I quit didn't I? Isn't that enough? Why can't I put on a little weight at the same time to reward myself? Yet, I know this is all my mind working me over and that I really don't want to put any weight on and I accept myself anyway."

"Even though food tastes so much better to me since I've quit smoking that I can't help myself from eating more food than I normally do, I love and accept myself nonetheless."

"Even though I want to eat more and food tastes better than it used to when I was smoking, I love and accept myself fully and completely nonetheless."

"I want to eat as much as I want. I want to eat sweets and special treats and experience as much satisfaction through food as I can since I don't smoke anymore. Yet, I know it's going to put more weight on me than I want and I know that's no good for me either and I accept myself, even if I never stop eating too much."

"I don't accept myself when I eat too much. I hate myself for not having enough self-control to stop eating when I know I've had enough and it's no longer any good for me. Yet, I love and accept myself fully and completely nonetheless."

"I hate myself when I over-eat and get out of control. I hate my body when it gets too fat and if it gets too fat from overeating, I'm afraid I might turn back to smoking if it means I won't have to be so fat and then everything I've worked so hard to achieve will fall flat on it's face. Yet, I love and accept myself fully and completely nonetheless."

"I can't stand the thought that I have so little self-control that I can't stop eating just like I stopped smoking. Yet, I love and accept myself fully and completely nonetheless."

"I wish I had more self-control over my eating. I'm so afraid I'm going to turn into a fat pig just because

I gave up smoking and that would never do. Yet I love and accept myself nonetheless."

"Ever since I stopped smoking, whenever I see food, I feel like I might get some measure of satisfaction that I'm missing since I stopped smoking. Yet, I know all the extra food is not helping me and I wish I could stop, but I feel powerless to stop and I accept myself nonetheless."

"I can't help myself when it comes to eating. I have no control at all. Yet, I love and accept myself fully and completely nonetheless."

"I'm completely lost when it comes to why I can't stop eating now that I've quit smoking. It's a complete mystery to me and it makes me feel so powerless, yet I love and accept myself fully and completely nonetheless."

"Even though I feel like I need to do something with my hands ever since I stopped smoking and that usually means I turn to handling food to make up for the cigarettes that I no longer handle, I love and accept myself fully and completely nonetheless."

"Even though I don't know what to do with myself when I have a drink without a cigarette, so I turn to filling my mouth with snacks and drinks instead and I know it's not doing me any good, I love and accept myself fully and completely nonetheless."

"Even though I don't know what to do with my hands when I don't have a cigarette in them and I often turn to food as a substitute and it's worrying me that I'm going to get fat, I love and accept myself fully and completely nonetheless."

"I feel like I'm completely at a loss of what to do about my mindless eating. I don't even notice that I've been eating until I'm completely stuffed and can't eat another bite and I'm already uncomfortable. Yet, I love and accept myself fully and completely nonetheless."

"Why can't I quit smoking without gaining weight? Why can't I muster the necessary willpower to eat less while I quit smoking? I just can't seem to do it. Yet, I love and accept myself nonetheless."

"I just can't seem to do it without outside help, but then I feel so incapable of handling my own eating habits and that frustrates me as well. Yet, I love and accept myself fully and completely nonetheless."

"I feel so powerless when it comes to food. It seems to control me more than I can control it. Yet, I love and accept myself fully and completely nonetheless."

"If I can't have a cigarette, which was always my one friend, then I should at least be allowed to eat whatever I want as a reward. So what if I get a little overweight? I love myself no matter what happens to me."

For those of you who are still having some difficulty in fully quitting smoking and want to use EFT to address those issues, here's a number of "bonus" wordings for you to use to finally stop smoking:

"I'm really afraid that I'm going to die of a heart attack if I don't stop smoking soon, yet I just can't seem to stop - no matter how hard I try. Yet, I love and accept myself full and completely nonetheless."

"I have a very serious heart (fill in yours) condition and know that my continued smoking is jeopardizing my health and my heart (fill in). Yet I just can't seem to stop smoking no matter how hard I try and I accept myself fully and completely nevertheless."

"If I don't stop smoking, I'm afraid I'll continue to do real damage to my heart and lungs and I'm really afraid of dying a painful and difficult death. Yet, despite everything I know and understand, I just can't stop smoking. Nevertheless, I'm doing the best I can and I accept and love myself."

"Even though I'm already having a lot of trouble breathing and a close relative of mine already has emphysema and I know I'm about to get it, if I don't already have it, I just can't seem to stop smoking no matter what I do. Yet, I love and accept myself fully and completely."

"Even though I know my body is no longer able to deal with all the terrible chemicals I'm putting into my body by smoking and I'm deathly afraid of getting cancer because of it, I just can't seem to quit no matter how hard I try. Yet I love and accept myself fully and completely no matter what happens to my body."

"Whenever I'm under stress of any kind, it doesn't matter how much fear of cancer or emphysema I have, I just have to have a cigarette and there's nothing I can do to stop that urge. Yet I love and accept myself fully and completely nonetheless."

"Why can't I give up this terrible habit of mine? Why do I keep smoking when I know it is so bad for me? I just haven't really been able to accept this change in my life yet, but I love and accept myself fully and completely nonetheless."

Here are some positive affirmations you can infuse after you've reached a zero in your SUDS scale on any issue, but especially about smoking. Say these positive affirmations as you tap on all the meridian access points one after the other:

> "I now know that I have fully given up my old smoking habit and I now choose to acknowledge that I'm no longer a smoker. In fact, I now realize that I'm a non-smoker for life and I appreciate that fact and feel proud of myself for making this change in my life."

> "I now choose to remain a non-smoker from this day forward for the rest of my life, knowing that it's the best thing that can happen to me and knowing that I can maintain this new way of being in the world without anxiety or stress accumulating within me."

> "I choose peace and happiness in my life, knowing that I'm entitled to it and knowing that I can maintain peace in my life from this day forward without having a cigarette ever again."

> "I choose to remain a non-smoker forever, knowing it will lead me to have a better, healthier life than ever before and I'm proud and pleased with my choices that led to this positive change in my life."

> "I am a non-smoker and I like how it feels."

> "I embrace being a non-smoker for life."

> "I like not spending all my money for it to go up in smoke."

> "I'm starting to feel better already and it can only get better."

> "I feel better now than I have in years."

"I like being able to climb a flight of stairs without suffering."

"I like not struggling to catch my breath all the time."

"I am starting to feel young again. I like that a lot."

"I'm feeling much better."

"I like being a non-smoker."

"I am now a non-smoker and know I'll be one for the rest of my life."

"This really is the first day of the rest of my life - as a non-smoker for life."

You may vary any of these positive affirmations in any fashion you wish so they more accurately reflect the ideas and thoughts you may have in your mind.

CHAPTER 2

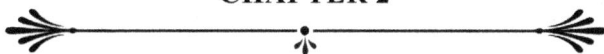

MAKE A MAJOR CHANGE IN YOU AND YOUR BODY

The following are some practical suggestions you can adopt at any time which will make a major change in you and your body. When you do them in conjunction with the previous suggestions about hypnosis and EFT, you'll discover that stopping smoking can actually lead you to becoming more conscious of your body and your mind and bring about major changes within you on many levels. In short, your life will improve dramatically in many ways once you stop smoking.

ALKALIZING YOUR BODY CHEMISTRY

When you smoke, you increase various acids in your body which result from the normal cellular process of your body. This is because by smoking, you clog up your lungs with tar and nicotine as well as 21 other dangerous chemicals. The normal exchange of gases (carbon dioxide and carbon monoxide with oxygen) that takes place in your lungs becomes impaired. Your body can't exhaust the ketone, acetone, lactic and other acids normally contained within the exhaled gases that result from the normal cellular processing of food used to convert the food to energy which the body utilizes for life.

Under normal conditions, when the cells of the body process food and sugars they produce certain chemicals and acids which are picked up by the hemoglobin in the blood and carried through the blood stream until it gets exhaled through the lungs. When this transition is made, there is an exchange of carbon dioxide and other gases for fresh oxygen that comes in through mouth and down into the lungs. The blood cells then transport the fresh oxygen that was picked up in the lungs to the cells in the body so they can use it produce more energy for the body's use and the process starts all over again.

When any part of this process is impaired (such as when the lungs are clogged with cigarette tar and other chemicals), the entire bodily process becomes impaired. When you use your lungs like a cigarette filter (which is effectively what they become when you smoke), they clog up and the normal exchange of oxygen and byproducts no longer occurs as it once did. The body then turns to other options. One of these options is to excrete those chemical byproducts and acids through the liver, kidney and eventually even through the skin. These organs are not as immediate or effective at eliminating acids from the body and the acids build up in these organs over time.

That's one of the reasons smokers are usually short of breath and don't have as much energy in their bodies. They have impaired their system by clogging it up with tar and other dangerous chemicals. It can't get the oxygen the cells need to operate normally and effectively.

However, one thing that is often overlooked is that the acids which are part of the byproducts of cellular activity tends to build up within the body which causes the Ph (which is the body chemistry scale between acid and alkalinity) to change and become more acidic. This can be very bad for your health.

In fact, it was discovered early in the 19th century that cancer flourishes in an acidic environment better than in any other environment. Perhaps this is why so many people who smoke eventually develop cancer in the lungs and many other areas of their bodies. That premise still remains to be proven by science, but statistics unequivocally show there is no doubt that smoking causes a higher incidence of cancer. It can occur in the lungs, but it also tends to show up in the lips, mouth, throat, nasal passages, gums, stomach, spleen, brain and a number of other places.

You can check your own Ph by buying some Ph strips at a drug store and checking it by following the directions for use. Remember, once you stop smoking, your body will probably need some time and attention to shift from an acidic chemistry to an alkaline chemistry. You can accomplish this change by introducing alkalizing foods and ionized water that will support such a shift in your body's Ph.

The most effective and natural process to alkalinizing your body is to introduce greens into your diet. Broccoli, brussels sprouts, kale, spinach, asparagus, collard greens, lettuce and other greens will help your body start to alkalize and there are a number of recipes in the back of this book to assist you in that direction.

HEALTHY DIET, EXERCISE AND MEDITATION

Dr. Dean Ornish, M.D. is a revered cardiologist who became well known as a "diet doctor" because of his focus over the past 25 years on showing people how they can change their bodies by changing their diets. Not by dieting! His book, Eat More, Weigh Less, is a fascinating read and is quite enlightening.

He actually became involved in this type of work because of his passion for cardiology and the fact that he noticed that so many people who went through heart bypasses and other cardiac procedures found themselves back in their doctor's offices within 3-5 years with the same cardiology issues despite their earlier surgeries.

He carefully studied a number of people and eventually came to the conclusion that heart surgery was not the panacea it was thought to be. He then came up with a combination of things that did prove to be successful at reconditioning the hearts of patients as old as 96 years of age. He recommends a change to a vegetarian diet, regular exercise and a combination of meditation and stress reduction that actually causes reversals in arterial congestion in people. And all this was **without** drug intervention. Just a healthy diet, exercise and meditation!

While he was initially attacked by the medical establishment for his controversial stand, they eventually realized he was onto something and embraced his findings. He's now well established as the authority in his field. We're going to give you an overview of his findings because they are actually encompassed within the context of the various suggestions offered in this book. We strongly suggest you read his books and get the full message directly from him.

First, he suggests that you <u>eliminate</u> red meat and dairy altogether. He also suggests that you become a vegetarian. Dr. Ornish found that by eliminating red mead and dairy in your diet, the bloodstream would become clearer and allow blood to flow better. He also found that by reducing stress, it reduces the blockages in the bloodstream. Interestingly enough, since the time that he originally wrote his first books on the topic, various studies have confirmed that stress, in and of itself, caused blockages within the bloodstream and that by reducing stress you can reduce those type of blockages. Other studies have also confirmed that smoking tends to lead to blockages in the bloodstream too.

He also suggests that a rudimentary exercise program is an integral and necessary part of regaining your health. He suggests regular cardiovascular exercise starting out with simple walking over short distances and then increasing the distance until you're walking at least a mile a day. As your health and stamina improve, you can progress to running if you want.

He also recommends yoga since it helps the body stretch and exercise simultaneously. Yoga can be practiced by anyone at any age and there are many forms of yoga from which to choose. He recommends that you enroll in a yoga studio and follow a format suggested and monitored by an instructor so you don't overdo it at the outset. You can try more challenging and complex yoga forms as you improve your physical fitness.

He also suggests many of the recommendations found later in this book. Eating at least 2 servings of fruits and vegetables at each meal and staying away from refined sugar are a great starting point to improve your cardiovascular health.

Dr. Ornish also suggests meditation, which is emptying the thinking part of the mind to achieve overall peace of mind. We suggest EFT in conjunction with meditation since we believe it enhances the meditative state once you eliminate everything that your mind is fixated on and directly helps you establish peace within your mind. In effect, its called Presence or becoming present. You can find out more about this valuable state of mind on our web site at hypno-eft.com and go to the Presence page. You can also discover more about Presence by visiting Leonard Jacobson's web site at leonardjacobson.com.

CHAPTER 3

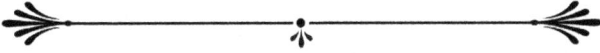

DIETARY RECOMMENDATIONS

Here are a number of practical suggestions for you to remain slim. By following them, you will also alkalize your body chemistry and markedly improve your health at the same time. You are not required to do any of them. They're simply recommendations offered to you to give you various ideas on how you can improve your health while you keep your weight down at the same time - as you stop smoking.

They are simple suggestions that are meant to give you a starting place so you can build on them in the future. Of course, you are free to amend or modify them to serve your own purposes, but by all means follow as many as possible and you'll soon notice you're only keeping the weight off, you're feeling better than you've felt in years.

1. Establish a Food Plan for Yourself in Advance. By making up a plan for the type of food you want to eat and for your meals the day before or even a week in advance, you will become more aware of everything you're going to eat. You'll be far less likely to stray from your plan and delve into the types of foods you know are not good for you. Everyone basically knows which foods they should be eating and which they should avoid. Yet, when we don't plan ahead, we often fall prey to whatever is in the refrigerator or our cupboards. Instead, set up a daily and weekly menu in which you lay out what you intend to eat and follow it as closely as possible. If you do this, you'll find you'll eat much healthier and take in far fewer fat and calories.

You'll also find you start to save money when food shopping because when you establish a Food Plan for your meals more than a day in advance, you'll be better able to establish a specific shopping list so that when you visit your supermarket, you're won't just be aimlessly walking around picking up whatever catches your eye. That will save you a lot of money in the long run and you will find you eat much healthier than you would if you just go with whatever interests you at the time you're shopping.

2. Eat Before You Shop. It is easier to avoid buying the wrong foods by eating <u>before</u> you go food shopping. If you go into a supermarket hungry, everything looks more attractive to you and you'll tend to buy far more of the wrong things than if you enter a grocery store with a full stomach and a specific shopping list.

3. Use a Food Journal. As you eat, enter everything you ate each day in a food journal to keep track of your daily intake. There's also no better way of becoming aware of what you've eaten than to have a list at the end of each day. At the end of each week, it's a good idea to review what you've eaten and stand on a scale and note your weight to see how much your weight has changed - if any. Nothing succeeds like success when it comes to taking weight off or keeping it off and nothing brings about greater mindfulness than constant vigilance.

4. Eat Breakfast. It's very important to start each day with breakfast. It gets your "motor" (metabolism) running, gives you a lot more energy to face the day and helps you use up what you eat better so there are no excess calories being stored as fat in your body by the end of the day. It also helps you eat less food throughout the day, especially if you include bran or other fiber-rich foods in your first meal of the day. Fiber takes longer to digest which means your blood sugar is less likely to spike right after that meal and will provide you with energy for a longer period of time as the body continues to digest it.

5. Go Slowly - But Keep on Going. If you're not comfortable with half your meal being vegetables or fruit, start out by adding just one fruit or vegetable serving a day. Then, as you get more comfortable with the taste and texture of fruits and vegetables, add another serving. Continue the process until you reach 8 to 10 servings a day. That's right, 8-10 servings a day. Every day. Of course, you can do 3-4 at each meal and or snack on vegetables to fill out the day's requirements. Carry around a small zip bag with baby carrots or celery and eat them as a snack. You can also carry around an apple or two along with an orange, tangerine or pear. Anything that is fresh and tasty will keep you energized, increase your fiber intake and not add a great number of calories to your intake.

6. Variety is Key. Eat at least two different servings of a fruit or vegetable at every meal. Yes, every meal. You'll find that as you start this process, you'll look forward to the fruits and vegetables as your taste for things change after you've quit smoking. The more you eat them, the better they taste.

7. Weigh yourself daily. While weekly weigh-ins are used by many well known weight loss programs, there are a number of studies that indicate that daily weigh-ins can make a big difference in levels of success and they are often the linchpin to permanent weight loss.

One study at the University of Minnesota discovered that of about 1,800 adults who were watching their weight carefully, those people who watched their weight daily lost twice as much weight as those who only stepped on a scale once a week.

Beyond that, those who weighed themselves daily were less likely to regain the weight they had lost. The simple act of stepping on the scale was enough to make a 100% difference in their weight loss and that's significant in anyone's book. One thing to remember is while there will be normal fluctuations in your weight, if it increases by more than 2-3 pounds in a week, it's a good time to stop eating desserts and other sweets and get back to basics again.

8. Eat with Purpose, Not Mindlessness. That means if you are eating, then think primarily about eating. If you're thinking about other things, then think of other things. but don't eat and think about other things at the same time. When you mix the two it will usually lead to mindless eating without noticing what you're putting in your mouth. That's why watching television while eating usually leads to obesity. Instead, whenever you eat, completely immerse yourself in the act of eating by using all of your senses of sight, smell, taste and touch to fully access the pleasure of nourishing your body - acknowledge the various tastes and smells that come with that nourishment.

Take the time to be fully present with your food, recognize you're taking this nutritious food into your body and it will supply you with energy throughout the day. Give thanks for it being there for you and for your body knowing how to use it effectively. In other words, take the time to enjoy your food fully. Make it an overall enjoyable experience, noticing everything about it and you will be surprised at how much better your food will taste and how much better it will serve you.

9. Beware of the Restaurant Trap. Never order more than you know you can eat while at any restaurant. Most diners and restaurants tend to make meals too large to begin with in order to justify their high prices. We tend to fall prey to those mammoth sizes at a "great price" and wind up eating far more than we should. Once you start to realize that their portions are too large, you may want to stop ordering the full dinners. Don't fall prey to ordering appetizers and extra plates just because they look tempting on the menu. Remember, just like your mother often told you, "your eyes are bigger than your stomach." Stay with smaller portions and eat slowly so you'll learn to recognize when your stomach is full. Stop before you eat everything on your plate and feel stuffed. You can always eat or order more if you really feel hungry at the end of your meal. Or you can stop eating earlier and take half of it home in a "doggie bag." Don't be embarrassed to take home half your meal. You paid for it. You deserve to enjoy it later if you wish.

10. Buddy System. Consider having a buddy system with a friend who is similarly working to stay slim or trim. Have meals together from time to time to talk about your progress. Each should have a food journal and you should enter each other's food intake when you're together. By making regular entries and reviewing it with your buddy regularly, you'll get a better idea of how honest you've been in your own food journal. This will help you become more conscious of how much and what you truly eat. You can also have some friendly competition with your buddy. Set goals from time to time and see who can accomplish them first. You can even wager home-cooked meals for fun.

11. Prepare Your Own Food. Don't rely upon prepared food items. There's a spiritual reason for this. When food is prepared by others who don't know or care about you, there's a disconnect between the food and its ultimate consumer. That disconnect is the simple fact that anyone could have prepared it (including a machine) and their energy could have "polluted" it. When such an energetic pollution strikes, you have no way of knowing about it ahead of time and no way of protecting yourself from it. Instead, prepare your own food or have someone who loves you and cares about you prepare it. Energetically, it will be much better for you and your higher consciousness will know the difference.

12. Maintain an 8-hour Workday as Much as Possible. Those who work overtime tend to put more weight on than those who work only 8 hours a day. In a study at the University of Helsinki, 7,000 adults were polled to see what their lifestyle was and whether it affected their weight. They discovered that those who had consistently worked overtime were far more prone to packing on the weight than those who stuck to a normal 8 hour work day. It appears that the contributing factors were a lack of time for normal meals and for exercise.

However, it was also an issue that most of those who worked overtime were under far more work-related stress than those who worked and left for home. That means that not only should you maintain your regular work schedule if possible, but if you find yourself under a great deal of stress, then it's time to introduce EFT into your life and reduce the stress - whether you work overtime or not. You'll feel much better and less stress means better health and the ability to maintain a more normal weight.

13. Sit down While You Eat (That Doesn't Mean Eating in Your Car While Driving). By sitting whenever you eat a meal, it affirms to your body and mind that it's time to eat and gives you a psychological break at the same time. It also automatically suggests that it's time to focus on eating and not two other things at the same time (such as driving and talking on the cell phone). That way, you'll start to digest your food as soon as you eat it rather than running around and trying to grab a bite of a sandwich in between driving, hammering nails or answering phones. It also gives you a little time to enjoy your food and reflect on what has transpired so far in your day and perhaps change the pace and direction of your day. It's also just good for you to sit down and eat. It honors you and your food as well.

14. Reduce Your Television Viewing to No More than 2 Hours a Day. Studies have conclusively shown that when you watch more than 2 hours of TV a day, you miss out on all the exercise you otherwise might have done. So if you reduce your television viewing to less than 2 hours a day, at least you'll get more exercise and you'll feel better at the same time.

Beyond that, it has also been shown that when people are sitting in front of a television, they tend to mindlessly eat more junk food than at any other time. So by limiting your time in front of the tube, you'll automatically limit your opportunity to eat that junk food that is so filled with calories, salt and so many other unhealthy substances.

One way to change this habit is to use a DVR Digital Video Recorder and tape all your shows so you can later watch them without all the commercials which are loaded with junk food suggestions. Not only will you use less time, you'll eliminate all those suggestive commercials at the same time.

Another thing you can do is place a sit-up chair, stationery bicycle or other exercise equipment in front of your television and exercise while you watch the video recordings of your favorite shows without the commercials or a DVD that you've brought home or downloaded from the Internet. All of these techniques will assist you in losing weight and allow you to exercise simultaneously.

SIMPLE WAYS TO REDUCE CALORIE INTAKE

The simplest solution is usually the best solution. The best way to hold down your weight is to reduce your calorie intake while making sure that you eat enough to power your body throughout the day. Eat less food. Eat the right food. Eat at the right times of the day.

15. Take it to Go. When eating out, cut any large portions in half and ask for the rest to be wrapped at the start of the meal to take home. Most diners and restaurant entrees contain between 1,500 and 2,000 calories and that's <u>without</u> the bread, butter, appetizer, sweetened beverage, or those beautiful, huge desserts.

Stay focused. Keep your eyes and mind open and don't overdo it just because you're in a restaurant and you can now afford it because you have extra money in your pocket because you've quit smoking. Eat half of what is on your plate and feel comfortable when you leave. That way, you'll have lunch the next day at no additional cost. There, you've not only saved money by not buying cigarettes, you've saved more money by taking half of your meal home for another day's meal. Not bad!

16. Proportion and Perception. Use a salad plate instead of a dinner plate to eat from. That way, whatever you eat will appear larger than if the same portion was on a huge plate. You'll also be less likely to unconsciously overeat because you're already making a choice to use a salad plate which brings your attention to what you're doing. You can ask for a salad plate even if you are eating out. Again, take whatever doesn't fit on the plate home and have it for lunch the next day. This may sound like a strange idea, but it actually works. It's amazing how we can deceive our minds when we choose to.

Are you starting to see a trend here? These are all methods of becoming more conscious of what you eat, when you eat and how much you eat, rather than allowing yourself to just fall into or remain in an unconscious fog every time you sit down to eat. That unconsciousness is what causes you to overeat in the first place and that's how many people start to put weight on in the first place.

17. Look at What You Eat. If your food is delivered in a bag at a fast food restaurant, ask for a paper plate and take the food out and put it on the plate so you can see how large your portion is <u>before</u> you start to eat it. That way, you'll be more conscious of how much food is available for you to eat. You'll find you're a lot less likely to just eat until everything is finished. Always eat slowly and put your attention on your stomach so that you'll notice as soon as you're starting to feel full. That way you can stop before you become stuffed and uncomfortable. This is an especially important habit to form and it will serve you well.

18. Start with the Most Filling Foods. Eat the lower calorie items on your plate first, like salad and vegetables, then move on to the meats, fish and eat your starches (like potatoes, bread, rolls, etc.) <u>last</u>. By the time you start eating them, you'll already be starting to feel full and you'll be better able to limit your intake of the highest calorie content parts of your meal. Plus, the vegetables and salad will be better able to start to be digested before the heavier parts of the meal descend upon them. Meats, fish and poultry don't digest as fast as vegetables, complex carbohydrates and starches. By eating in this fashion, you'll find you will start to lose weight effortlessly.

19. Fat is Fat. Whole milk is higher in butter fat content than skim milk, but fat is fat, regardless of its source. It's best to avoid milk altogether once you're no longer a child.

Here's a way to make the switch from milk smoothly. First, switch from whole milk to 1 or 2 percent milk. It may initially taste a little thin, but after a couple of days it will become normal to you. You'll then find that after a couple of weeks, you won't want to go back to whole milk. Remember, just by drinking a glass of reduced fat milk a day, you'll naturally lose about 5 lbs. in a year over drinking the same amount of whole milk. Five Pounds!

Better than that, once you've switched to skim milk, then you can eventually switch to rice milk, almond or soy milk. They may not sound so great to you at first, but once you drink any of them for a few days to a week, 1-2% milk will taste and feel as heavy by comparison as whole milk did to skim milk. After that the other "milks" will help you make a similar transition. You'll lose even more weight with them than with the reduced fat milk and you'll develop less phlegm than with any type of cow's milk derivative. Almond milk now that has no sugar in it at all and no fat content and it tastes great.

20. Avoid Juices. Fruit juices contain a lot of calories. They usually have more calories than soda and while they're better than soda, it would be best to set a limit of one glass a day. If you want to drink more than one glass of juice a day, try diluting each glass by 1/3 with water which will automatically reduce your caloric intake by a similar amount.

21. Avoid Diet Soda. Avoid drinking <u>all diet sodas</u> since it's been repeatedly reported that their sweeteners will ultimately lead to higher caloric intake and many have been linked to cancer and other health problems. The sweeteners also usually leave a bad taste in your mouth but most people get used to it because the idea of zero calories is so attractive. What they don't usually notice is the increase in food they eat after they've been drinking a diet soda for awhile. Whether it's to ease the bad aftertaste or for some other reason, most people who regularly drink diet sodas find they don't lose weight by doing so. Instead, they either stay the same or gain weight while drinking them.

The second issue is that low calorie soda sweeteners tend to be somewhat carcinogenic, a fact that's been proven by many studies. It's usually only been the case when the sweetener or the soda within which it's contained is exposed to high temperatures for any length of time. The problem with this is, when you buy a soda, it's usually chilled and there's no way of knowing if it's been previously exposed to high temperatures before you drank it. It's probably a safer bet to leave it alone and stay with water or diluted fruit juices.

22. Drink about 8 Glasses of Water Each Day. Water can increase your body's metabolism. German researchers discovered that by drinking two 8-ounce glasses of <u>cold</u> water it increased people's metabolic rate by as much as 30% for a short period of time. Interestingly, the effect lasted for over an hour. That means that anything you eat at the same time will be metabolized by your body at a higher rate than with room temperature water. Another interesting fact was that fully one-third of the metabolic boost came from warming the water within the body. The rest of the metabolic boost came from the absorption by the body of the water. Just by drinking water you are using additional calories, unlike when you drink any other fluid that has caloric content, such as iced tea, soda and fruit juices. If you want to lose weight easily and effortlessly, start drinking water before you eat every meal and every snack and if you want to increase your metabolism, drink cold water.

23. Share Dessert. When eating out and you're checking out the dessert tray or display case in the dinner, make sure you only order <u>one</u> dessert and <u>two</u> or <u>three</u> spoons and plates for the entire table. Share it with family members and divide the calories among all of you rather than pigging out alone or buying more than one dessert. Everyone will be happier on the ride home and you'll all have the same memory to share of that wonderful dessert. Just less of it. It also brings out a feeling of family or community when you share with one another.

24. Eat Only until You're about 3/4 Full. The rest will take care of itself. This may sound like a cliche, but it works! It takes you about 20 minutes to get the signal that you are full from your stomach.   When you're not fully conscious of the fullness of your stomach, you're more likely to overfill it before you realize it.

Remember every Thanksgiving dinner you've ever had? Remember sitting on the sofa watching football and lamenting about overeating as your stomach aches?

Instead, only eat about 3/4 of what you think you should be eating and stop. Then evaluate how your stomach feels. If you feel full, stop eating. If not, go right ahead and keep on shoveling it in.

You'll be surprised at how effective this simple technique can be at eliminating more than 1/4 of what you eat and never really enjoyed. In fact, as you become more conscious of how much you're eating, you'll notice that you will usually save even more than 1/4 of the food you would have unconsciously eaten. And you'll feel better for it.

25. Go for the Lower Calorie Alternative. Substitute mustard for mayonnaise on sandwiches whenever possible. Mayonnaise is made of oil and eggs. Both are high in fats and calories. Mustard is a great substitute, has far fewer calories and has a great and zesty taste. Granted, it takes some getting used to the new taste at first, but once you do, it's actually a great taste treat. There are a number of different types of mustard on the store's shelves and there are more specialty mustards than ever before. Try a few until you find the precise taste that you enjoy the most with each type of food. As you do, you'll find you're losing weight and enjoying your food more.

26. Eat More Soup. Eat broth-based soups, not cream-based. Creamy soups add too many calories and too much fat content, neither of which will help your cause. Try soups with lots of vegetables, you'll naturally reduce your calories and increase your fiber intake. If you buy your soup canned, make sure to read the labels to see what ingredients are used in making the soup. Try to look for soups with less ingredients and watch the salt content. Its no good for your heart and your blood pressure. Try to avoid soups made with ingredients you can't pronounce, that's always a good bet that it will be healthier for you.

27. Reduce Your Intake of Soda, Sweetened Iced Tea and Other Sweetened Drinks. Here's another reason to avoid them. Almost every one of them has a high sugar content which not only adds unnecessary calories, but is also harmful to your body. That's primarily because the sugars used are refined sugar rather than natural sugars. Instead, substitute water or reduced sugar drinks. You may also wish to substitute stevia or other natural sugar substitutes for sugar. However, <u>don't</u> drink low calorie or diet drinks since they usually contain aspartame or other carcinogenic ingredients which can change your metabolism and are inherently dangerous.

28. Bring Your Lunch to Work. First, it's cheaper. It's also easier to plan what you're going to eat ahead of time and you can plan exactly what you're going to eat. You'll enjoy it more because you get to choose what you eat by what you bring. You'll also find that you can eat much better food by bringing whatever you want rather than settling on whatever is available at the local Deli, fast food store or one of those "Deli trucks."

29. Get Most of Your Calories from Foods You Chew, Rather than Commercially Prepared Beverages. Beverages are largely processed food which have been crushed, filtered and have preservatives in them to maintain their "freshness." You never know how long they've been sitting on a truck in the hot sun or sitting on a shelf or in a box before you bought it. Instead, have fresh fruit or freshly squeezed fruit juice whenever you can. It contains pulp which contains fiber which takes longer to digest so your body will have a more constant sugar level and that means more energy over a longer period of time for you. While you're chewing, you're adding your own bodily juices to begin the digestive process so by the time it reaches your stomach the process is already well underway. Most importantly, fresh fruit tastes better and is better for you. Make the effort to eat fresh and eat organic whenever you can. You'll be rewarded with better health and greater enjoyment.

30. Eat at Home Rather than at Restaurants. By eating at home, you'll save money on food and be able to eat better food or determine exactly what you want rather than just what's on the menu. You'll also get to plan your meals in advance and save money. It's always fun and enjoyable to eat out and not have to prepare food and wash the dishes, pots and pans afterward, but do it as a rare treat. That way, you'll appreciate it more.

Also, by eating at home, you'll also be able to get organic fruits and vegetables into your diet at very little extra cost. Another thing that most people don't often think about - when your food is prepared at home, it is prepared by people (yourself included) that care about what they're doing and usually prepare it with love. That can make a big energetic difference from food prepared by strangers who don't know you or care about you.

31. Limit or Eliminate Alcohol. If you choose to continue to drink alcohol, reduce your alcohol intake to weekends with the goal of eventually eliminating it altogether. Not only is alcohol very high in calories, it puts a tremendous strain on your body, especially your liver and kidneys, to say nothing of the brain cells it kills each time you imbibe. Alcohol also appears to "burns hotter" in your body than normal food and that's why after you've been drinking you will often wake up in the middle of the night with a dreadfully dry mouth or in a sweat. The water in your system has been "burned off" by the higher rate of metabolism and you need to fill your tank again.

Of course, that's not good for the body either since it's best to always remain fully hydrated. It's best to eliminate alcohol from your life if possible, other than for an occasional glass of wine or beer with a meal. It appears that when you have a glass of wine or beer with a meal it allows the body to metabolize it simultaneously and smooths out the process so you don't normally get that adverse level of bodily response as when you just drink alcohol alone.

See the Appendix for the amount of calories in each type of major drink. It should help you better understand and appreciate what you're drinking so you can have a good time and not gain too much weight as you enjoy yourself.

EAT MORE VEGETABLES

"What do I do if you don't want to eat vegetables?" This is a common concern for many people. Beyond saying "get over it," the first thing to remember is that vegetables are the best means to alkalize your body chemistry, maintain your blood sugar at a healthy level and provide the nutrients needed to sustain your life. The vitamins, enzymes and fiber contained in vegetables are well worth their weight in gold when it comes to insuring your health.

While you can take vitamin supplements, they are never as good as the real thing. Vegetables may not always the most tantalizing taste treats by themselves, but if you add spices and flavorings that alter their plain and sometimes bitter taste, you'll be quite surprised at how good they can taste. Sometimes it takes being a good cook to make them taste better. Here are some additional suggestions to help you make them taste better and find ways of eating vegetables in different ways that may pleasantly surprise you.

32. Load Up on Vegetables. When eating at a restaurant, order a salad first and finish it before ordering anything else. That way, you'll already be nearly full and somewhat satisfied before you even consider ordering an entree. You'll be less prone to over-ordering and overeating. Again, always eat each course slowly and notice when your stomach starts to feel full. You'll stop eating earlier, save yourself from taking in a lot more calories and take more food home with you for the next day. Likewise, when eating at home, start with a salad before you start your main course and take your time eating it so you will feel full before you start to dole out your main meal.

33. Vegetables and Fruits. Again, make sure your plate is half vegetables and/or fruit at both lunch and dinner. Add a salad of fresh uncooked vegetables to your meal and you'll notice a difference. You can also add cut up fresh fruit or canned mandarin orange segments that have been thoroughly drained to a salad to make it sweeter, more tasty and more interesting. You can also add fresh broccoli, cauliflower or fresh leafy greens like spinach or kale as a side dish or part of your evening meal. These will also give you additional roughage and add to your overall intake of green leafy vegetables to help alkalize your body chemistry.

34. Have More Raw Vegetables at Each Meal, but Especially at Lunch. You'll find that the fiber in raw foods will stay with you much longer than processed or cooked foods so you won't get hungry as quickly and your blood sugar will remain more consistent for longer periods of time throughout the day. This will help you eliminate those sugar lows in the middle of the afternoon. Many people snack to fill that energy gap, and often choose the wrong foods because it's the only thing available in the vending machine. By eating foods filled with fiber and roughage, the body takes longer to digest them and therefore, your blood sugar stays at a more even level for longer periods of time.

35. Vegetable Juice. One way to get more "vegetables" into your system is to have vegetable juice or even a can of V8 if you can't make your own fresh vegetable juice. It's convenient and it's filled with eight varieties of vegetables and it's a great substitute for soda or even fruit juice. If you keep the juice chilled, it tastes quite refreshing. Again, because of the fiber content, vegetable juice will give you a longer burst of energy than juice or soda.

36. Season and Flavor Your Vegetables. Make your vegetables more palatable by adding things to them like seasoning (cinnamon, nutmeg, pepper, paprika, oregano, etc.- NOT salt), nuts, raisins, dried cranberries, blueberries or other dried fruit like sliced apricots or mangos. You'll be surprised at how much flavor fresh or dried fruits will add to your vegetables and how it can change the way they taste. By adding dried fruits and nuts to your vegetables, you also improve how they are visually presented on a dish or plate. Try them, you'll like them

37. Use Beans for Protein. Mix different varieties of rinsed, drained canned beans for a high protein salad. You may wish to use vinegar based dressing since it is good for your body and low in calories. A prepared salad of this type will usually keep well for about a week or more in your refrigerator. This is an excellent way to get some additional protein into your food plan without eating more meat. Its high fiber content also helps with digestion and elimination which is important to your health.

38. Vegetable Soup. If you make your own hearty soup at home in advance, make sure to include fresh vegetables such as carrots, beets, broccoli, potatoes, peppers, onions, beans, peas, spinach, kale, chives, and especially any other green leafy types that will help you alkalize your body chemistry and you'll also avoid preservatives that canned soups usually have in them. If you make it thick like a stew, it will be more filling and not high in calories since it will be mostly vegetables.

39. Baked Potato <u>Without</u> Sour Cream or Butter. Add <u>mustard</u> instead. It takes a little getting used to the new taste at first, but once you do, you'll immediately notice the difference in how you feel and how you start to look. It will make a difference by reducing your caloric and fat intake as soon as you eliminate the butter and sour cream. Plus, mustard isn't as filling as when you eat potatoes with butter or sour cream. Potatoes can be a great source of more than just complex carbohydrates and they taste good at the same time.

40. Try a Sweet Potato. Bake a sweet potato and add a little cinnamon to taste if needed. Sweet potatoes are a tasty treat and are loaded with more fiber than regular potatoes. Without the butter, you'll also notice a distinct difference in caloric and fat intake and you'll get to taste the sweet potato even better. If you absolutely need that buttery taste, use a butter substitute.

41. Use Baby Spinach in New Ways. You can add it to sandwiches instead of iceberg lettuce (which has no nutritional value in it) and have them in salad. You can also add it to pasta or eat it by itself pan-fried with olive oil, garlic and herbs such as chives, oregano or thyme. Baby spinach is filled with minerals like iron and will usually help you become more regular in your elimination process.

42. Join a Food Cooperative. Get the best organic food available at the best prices. It may take a little bit of your time and/or money (they usually ask you to donate some of your time to man the store or donate some money if you don't work), but it's well worth it in the long run. The food is usually excellent and most of it is often organic. You'll also find healthier choices for everything from pet food to household cleansers and personal items. You'll also be part of a community that is concerned with health not only for their families but for the environment.

43. Use Emotional Freedom Technique. Yes, EFT. For some, aversion to vegetables may come from an early event in your personal history such as being told you can't leave the table until you finish all your spinach, etc. That can leave a negative association and keep you from enjoying a great vegetable that helps you alkalize your body chemistry. Rather than just trying to hold your nose and eating vegetables that you don't like, try EFT to tap the issue away. You can do it for any vegetable or anything else you don't want to eat and see how much more you enjoy your meals afterward.

Just tap on the various meridian access points (you can find them in the diagram in the Appendix) while saying words like, "Even though I don't want to eat this (spinach, broccoli, cauliflower, brussels sprouts, etc. - whatever it is you dislike), I love and accept myself anyway." Then tap on each meridian access point while saying, "This spinach; I hate broccoli; I can't stand cauliflower, etc." Do one vegetable at a time and before long, your distaste for each vegetable will evaporate and you'll find that you start to enjoy them. If you don't yet know how to do EFT, review the EFT chapter for a full explanation and you can always go to our web site at hypno-eft.com and click on the EFT page and you'll find free videos, a full description and a downloadable diagram that you can follow. While EFT may look a bit weird at first, it really works and it works well to eliminate negative thoughts, self-limiting beliefs as well as pain.

44. Frozen Vegetables. Keep various frozen vegetables in your freezer and mix and match them for variety. You can keep bags of peas, carrots, potatoes, broccoli, string beans, etc. and change the mixture each day until you find a combination you especially like. Then, the next week start all over again and find a new mixture that you like. You can add different types of soup or stock for flavor or you can add different spices such as garlic, oregano, paprika, thyme, pepper and even cinnamon. You can also use different vinegar based salad dressings or add a bit of fruit such as mandarin orange slices or canned pears (both should be drained first) for a pleasant change of pace. You can add fresh fruit such as sliced mango, peaches, apples and any number of other alternatives.

CHANGE YOUR FOOD INTAKE AND
IMPROVE YOUR HEALTH

By ending your smoking habit, you've taken a giant step forward in regaining your health. By changing your diet at the same time, you can not only change the Ph in your body, you can improve your health at the same time. By eliminating excess fats, complex carbohydrates and refined sugar from your diet while you add green leafy vegetables to it, you will be making a world of difference to your body and its chemistry. Here are some practical ideas on how to change your eating habits as well as what you eat so your health will improve.

45. Eat Healthy Snacks. Whenever you feel a mid-afternoon emotional or energy low, it's usually because your blood sugar is running low. Instead of having that extra cup of coffee or caffeine drink as a pick-me-up, have a V8 juice, a fresh vegetable snack or a yogurt instead. The fiber in the vegetables, which take longer to digest, will carry you through to dinner with no added caffeine and you'll feel better for it in both your body and your mind in the long run.

Also, while caffeine works wonders to juice up your attention almost immediately and gives you the feeling of having more energy, it also has a down side to it that leaves you feeling worse after the initial high wears off. Of course, you could put that off by having another cup of coffee, but that only makes the eventuality of the down side worse. The better approach is to limit your coffee and caffeine intake to one cup a day (two at most) to maintain a solid balance of internal energy without the inevitable lows that accompany caffeine.

46. Prepare Snacks in Advance. If you're energy level is waning at mid-morning or by 3-4 p.m. at work and there are no healthy snacks available, bring your own snacks like almonds or other nuts in a small plastic bag or container and carry them with you. They're good for you and tasty at the same time. Add dried fruits like cranberries, blueberries, raisins or apricots for taste, and you'll start to look forward to a healthy snack instead of whatever is in the vending machine. Nuts take longer to digest so they will maintain your blood sugar in a more consistent manner and will last in your body better than sweet processed foods.

47. Don't Ever Skip Breakfast. Eat a healthy breakfast filled with antioxidants and complex carbohydrates. Things like whole grain cereals and breads, berries and fruit. It doesn't take long and it's well worth it. You may wish to start with a fresh fruit smoothie in a blender using a cup of plain or vanilla yogurt, frozen blueberries, strawberries, a banana and pealed kiwi. Add ice to thin it out if you want. It makes a 2-cup serving which has under 350 calories and is very low in fat. It tastes great and is good for you. You can also take it on the road easily which saves time later if you commute. See the end of the book for more smoothie recipes.

48. If You Need to Use Oil, Use Olive Oil. If you use butter, corn or peanut oil to cook, replace them with olive oil. It's the only type of oil that doesn't deteriorate under heat. Do your best not to cook with any oils if you can, since they all change dramatically for the worse to some extent when you heat them. This advice might lead many people to think of using Teflon or other stick-free pans, but that's not the answer either. There have been reports that non-stick surfaces can be carcinogenic. Instead, use quality stainless steel pans and cook at lower heats for longer periods of time and watch your food carefully. If you closely monitor whatever you're cooking and turn it often, it won't stick or burn. Its well worth the effort.

49. Use Apple Sauce Instead of Butter or Oil. That's right. You can use unsweetened apple sauce instead of the normal amount of butter that any recipe calls for and you'll enjoy a moist, fatless outcome. This works especially well with brownies if you're making them from scratch or if the store bought recipe calls for the addition of a tablespoon of butter, then you can add two tablespoons of applesauce instead and you should get about the same consistency in the finished brownie with no fat content. You may have to experiment a little with the amount of applesauce to use in each type of recipe, but you'll definitely enjoy the outcome knowing there is no fat content when you're done.

50. Whole Wheat. Use whole wheat flour instead of white flour when making bread, rolls, muffins, pancakes or anything else whenever you can. It will make a big difference in your digestion and it increases the amount of fiber you take into your system. By adding fiber to your intake, it helps your digestion and elimination processes. As we've repeatedly mentioned, fiber helps your food "last longer" so that you don't run out of energy as fast as you will with white flour products.

51. Eliminate All Cold Cuts and Deli Meats from Your Diet. They are packed with salt (which helps your body retain water and gain weight) and other chemicals and preservatives to keep them from rotting while they sit in the deli display case for weeks on end. Also, remember that bologna and other mixed types of deli meats are made from an assortment of meat and other animal <u>parts</u> and spices and some even include <u>chicken feet</u> that have been ground up. Instead, replace them with fresh sliced turkey breast, and lean fresh roast beef if you eat red meat or you can also use tuna or chicken salads instead of deli meats.

52. Peanut Butters. In recent tests, brand name peanut butters like Skippy, JIF and Peter Pan were determined to have levels of trans fats lower than .5 gram per 2-tablespoon serving. They also contained only 1 gram more sugar than natural brands, which is an insignificant difference. However, if you want to be really sure of a natural product, you can use natural peanut butter and stir it up each time you use it.

53. Other Nut Butters. Consider almond butter, cashew or other nut butters since they each have a different chemistry than peanut butter and different tastes that will give you variety and healthful benefit's at the same time. Most of them don't use any trans fats and need to be stirred to use them, but they taste good and they're good for you.

HEALTHY EATING WITHOUT ALL THE COOKING

Many people like to eat food but don't especially like to cook it or clean up after cooking and eating it. If you're one of them, here are a number of alternative ideas that will help you continue to eat healthily while at the same time not forcing you to cook. Of course, there's always some cleanup involved, but at least you won't feel like you're slaving over a hot stove in the middle of a hot summer when you follow these suggestions.

54. Remember That Smoothie. You can make it with fat-free milk, soy or almond milk, fresh fruit, frozen fruit, and add some wheat germ for more substance. Also, consider adding some Greens+ green powder for green vegetable content. See the recipes at the end of the book for many alternatives.

55. Vegetarian Takeout. Try a vegetarian Thai or Chinese food take out meal and green tea, which is often included free with the meal. Take it home to enjoy and then, as dessert, have a piece of fruit, some baby carrots, a small custard or a live culture yogurt afterward to round out the meal and make it even healthier. Make sure you order your meal so that it doesn't have MSG (monosodium glutamate) in it which can have a very negative effect on many people. If you already have heart or weight problems, tell them not to use salt either. Obviously it's best to not eat Chinese take out every night, however, once in a while can be a treat.

56. Peanut Butter and No-Sugar-Added Jelly. Consider a peanut butter and no-sugar jelly (called fruit-only preserve) sandwich on whole wheat bread with a glass of soy, almond or rice milk, or even maybe some 1 percent milk and a piece of fruit like an apple, orange or tangerine. You may also wish to put the peanut butter and no-sugar jelly on crackers or a rice cake for a different taste and texture.

57. Shortcuts. Bake or broil (microwave only if you must) frozen pre-cooked chicken strips and frozen broccoli or peas topped with mustard sauce or a clear dressing like Balsamic vinegar and olive oil. It's quick and easy to make and is low in calories and fat content.

58. Pre-Made. Bake a healthy frozen dinner entree and add a fresh spring salad with a clear dressing such as Balsamic vinegar and olive oil or a low fat prepared clear dressing, along with a cup of green tea or flavored herbal tea. Stay away from creamy dressings as they are high in both calories and fat content.

59. Breakfast for Dinner. Scramble eggs in a stainless steel skillet (not a stick free surface - it's been discovered that they're not great for you). Pop some cut up asparagus in at the end just as the eggs are almost done, and add dry whole wheat toast to the dish. If your cholesterol levels are normal, you can have eggs almost every day. They're good for you, high in protein and are a good energy source. If your cholesterol isn't what it should be, you may want to try an egg white omelette from time to time. However, don't be afraid of whole eggs, they can actually help reduce your cholesterol. Try different flavorings other than ketchup, such as mustard, horseradish, ginger, fresh pepper, onions, garlic, etc. to add a different touch to your dish. Also, add a little interesting garnish such as greens and tomatoes for color and a different taste.

60. Pre-Packed Salad. Use a pre-packaged salad (there are many varieties available), topped with drained canned tuna, salmon, chicken or fresh turkey. Add some grape tomatoes and a clear type dressing and you have a nice meal that is low in fat and calories. If you feel you must have something more solid, try adding some low fat crackers to the meal.

61. Make a Healthy Sandwich. Keep healthy sandwich ingredients around the house, including whole wheat bread and whole wheat crackers. Also make sure to have sliced organically raised or free range turkey or chicken, tomatoes and mustard or low fat mayonnaise with horseradish made into a sauce kept in the refrigerator.

62. Low Salt, Preservative Free Canned Soups. Heat up a can of healthy soup or even noodle soup and add a variety of fresh cut vegetables to fill out the meal and have some low fat crackers on the side. Add a cup of herbal tea and you have a warm and enjoyable meal for very little cost which takes very little work.

63. Eat Healthy at Fast Food Restaurants. Try a veggie sandwich or salad at a fast food restaurant. They're getting better and better. Make sure to leave out the croutons and noodles. The natural fiber in the meal will keep your blood sugar consistently high for hours unlike a normal fast food meal.

AVOID OVEREATING DURING
THE HOLIDAYS, SPECIAL EVENTS AND PARTIES

Almost everybody looks forward to the holidays when family and friends get together to share the joy of "the most wonderful time of the year." It's usually at those times that our defenses are lowered and we act out like the kids we are at heart as we regress right back to being that little kid looking for something to give them comfort.

We often reach for the very foods that gave us the most comfort when we were young and before we know it, we're overeating and wondering why we put on so much weight over the holidays.

Another scenario is we sit down at the table and eat everything in sight because "that's what you're supposed to do," isn't it? Then we wind up uncomfortably sitting on the sofa as we open up our pants and watch football. Either way, it not only packs the pounds on, it is unhealthy and will undo everything you accomplished in the weeks and months leading up to the holidays.

Instead, if you keep your wits about you and don't regress too badly and perhaps even prepare in advance for the potential problems that could arise, you have a good chance of overcoming the usual rituals of over-eating that often accompany the holidays.

Here are some practical tips to help you get through the holiday season comfortably so you can emerge on the other side feeling as slim and in control as you were before they started.

64. It's Not OK. First, don't rationalize that it's "okay" to eat everything in sight just because "it's Thanksgiving" or one of the other holidays. Of course, allow yourself some latitude in what and how much you eat, but maintain your new conscious eating style throughout all the holidays and you'll appreciate it later and feel better about yourself.

65. Don't Eat Emotionally. Use EFT. The rational mind can make up just about any excuse to justify anything and especially when you're eating all of your comfort foods during the holidays. That's when all the old family issues have a way of arising again as they did when you were a child. It's amazing how seeing family members who you don't see most of the year can bring up old "stuff" and make you feel emotionally uncomfortable. That's when you're most vulnerable and most likely to "fall off the wagon" or eat or drink uncontrollably in an attempt to feel better or more comfortable.

However, if you realize in advance that this is likely to happen to you, you'll be a lot better able to deal with it if it arises by resolving it in advance. First, be more conscious of your inner feelings and watch when any insecurities arise within you regarding the upcoming holidays and/or your family so you can use EFT to deal with them when they arise. The best time to eliminate them easily and completely is as they initially arise within you. As soon as you feel the least bit uncomfortable, excuse yourself and go to the bathroom or somewhere else and tap all the meridian access points and focus your wording on what made you uncomfortable. It usually works quickly and easily and eliminates those negative feelings so you can go back to your family and friends without all the stress you were feeling just minutes before.

Once the old feelings are gone, you'll find it is much easier to deal with anything else that may arise as you go along. Here are a few ideas and wording suggestions that will help you through the rest.

Use EFT to tap on the issue:

> "Even though I hate it when everyone starts talking about what I was like when we were young and it gives me a lot of stress and then I reach out for comfort food or alcohol and I get carried away and

the next thing I know I'm packing on the pounds. Yet I love and accept myself and my insecurities."

"Even though I hate going to family events because I always feel so uncomfortable and it usually leads me to drink and eat to excess and then I feel even more uncomfortable. Yet, I'm doing the best I can and that will have to do for now."

"Even though I want to be like everyone else and eat as much as I want at parties and dinners, I seem to lose all control once I start eating and wind up putting on weight. Yet, I love and accept myself nonetheless."

"Whenever I am around my family my old insecurities come back to haunt me and I feel so terrible whenever anyone says anything to me, so I turn to my comfort food and satisfy my needs by eating more than I should and then I feel terrible because I'm afraid of putting weight on again after working so hard to take it off. Yet I love and accept myself no matter what happens."

Remember to use words and meanings from the Set-Up phrases as Reminder phrases as you tap on all the meridian access points since they help you keep your mind focused on the issue. They might sound like this:

EB - "I'm under so much pressure at family gatherings."
SE - "I just can't take it anymore."
UE - "I feel so insecure around my family."
UN - "I hate the holidays."
UM - "Holidays are very difficult for me."
CB - "I wish my family was different towards me."
UA - "I always tend to turn to food for comfort."
TH - "I really want to change all this but feel helpless."

Change the "reminder phrases" to fit your specific issues and whatever you're tapping on at the time so they are consistent with your intent.

66. Never Go to a Party Hungry. Some people think the whole idea of going to a party where food will be served is to stuff their face and drink as much as possible because "it's on the house.". Usually they are grossly overweight and still wondering why. Avoid that trap. If you're hungry before a party, it's always best to eat a little something just before you leave your house to go to the party so you won't be prone to mindless overeating. Eat an apple, yogurt, nuts, carrots, etc. to give you an energy lift before getting to the party where there will probably not be as many healthy things for you to eat. Also, by eating beforehand, if you have an alcoholic drink, you won't be as prone to getting intoxicated and losing your original intent to not overeat or over drink. By following this simple plan, you'll be better able to keep your positive eating practices intact and wake up the next morning feeling good about yourself rather than feeling foggy from overeating or over-drinking the night before.

67. Stay Away from the Food Table. Literally avoid standing near the food table at parties. Purposely pick a spot on the opposite end of the room or in another room where there is no food and stay there as much of the night as possible. That doesn't mean to stand at the bar either. Remember, out of sight, out of mind. It works. Now take a moment to consciously affirm that this is a great idea for you and vow to do it the next time you're at a party. Also take a deep breath and internalize your new intent.

68. Don't Graze. If a buffet is offered, instead of grazing like most people do, choose just a few items you like and eat just what you chose. And don't go back for seconds. Otherwise, you'll find yourself more tempted by everything else and eating far more than you ever expected. Again, if you do graze, you'll more than likely wake up the next morning filled with regret and a bulging belly.

69. Don't Leave Room to Grow Into Your Clothes. Throughout the holidays, wear the tightest clothes you have. They won't allow you any room for expansion. That's right, make sure you must open that top button on your pants whenever you overeat. It will make you more conscious of your body when you're feeling fat or it will make you worried that your clothing is going to split open at every seam whenever you overeat. It's a great incentive to become mindful of every bite you put into your mouth. That way, you'll be more prone to eat less and keep your figure intact throughout the holidays. Avoid wearing sweats suit's altogether until March (at least until after the Super Bowl is over).

70. Share the Wealth. Before your guests leave, give them all the leftovers you have from the food table. That way there's no extra food hanging around just waiting to be eaten by you and your guests will be happy to take their favorite dish home with them. It's a win-win situation for everyone.

EXERCISE IS A NECESSITY

While it's wonderful that you've chosen to be more mindful of what you eat, the other component to staying slim while you stop smoking is to increase the amount of exercise you do.

Doing aerobic exercise means you get your heart rate up and keep it elevated for at least twenty minutes. You can do this by briskly walking, running, stair climbing, dancing, making love, doing calisthenics or any number of other ways to keep your heart pumping fairly rapidly for a prolonged period. When you do it enough over a long enough period, your body and heart will adapt and that will make you healthier. It also appears to clean out your arteries because your blood is rushing through them and flushing them out due to all the physical exertion.

Anaerobic exercise is using your muscles to lift or move different objects that have some weight to them, causes your muscles to increase in size as you increase the repetitions or weight of the barbells or other items you may use.

We suggest you do both aerobic and anaerobic exercises. That way, you will not only increase your heart rate which is great for every part of your body, you will also tone your muscles at the same time. By doing this you will naturally increase your body's metabolism and once it's been increased, it will effectively burn off any extra calories that might have otherwise turned into fat.

What happens when you take in more calories in your food and drink than you need to function is it turns into fat, which is really just stored energy. Whatever is turned into fat is intended by the body for future use whenever its needed by the body. If it never gets used, it remains in the body as stored energy and in this case stored energy makes you look and feel fat.

Here are some simple and practical suggestions on how you can incorporate exercise into your daily regimen and feel much better because of it.

71. Make Exercise a Daily Priority. No excuses. Do it. You'll feel better and look better for it. You don't have to do an hour a day. Start with five or ten minutes of plain calisthenics (pushups, sit-ups, deep knee bends, etc.) and walking and work up from there. You'll feel better about yourself and your body as each day goes by. It won't be long until you turn that ten minutes into twenty and later even more. Exercise is a good thing to get addicted to at any age.

72. Dance! Start dancing at home with your family. It may sound strange, but it works once you start doing it. Start watching "Dancing with the Stars" which has been a big incentive for many people in America and other parts of the world like England and Australia to start ballroom dancing. It gives the entire family something to do together and you'll all get healthier by doing it regularly.

73. Walk Before You Shop. Walk around the mall at a fast pace three times before you start shopping. That way, you'll get in a substantial amount of exercise beforehand and also locate where the sales are before you start shopping. It's amazing how effective this can be for you because by exercising you'll also dissipate any stress you had in your body and mind and you'll find you're that much less inclined to buy things that you don't need and you'd normally buy as a response to stress. The mall is also a great place to exercise during inclement weather and throughout the winter months when it may be too cold outside to exercise outdoors. Or for those in southern climates, it's a great place to exercise when its too warm outside during the summer months. Either way it works great and is something you should do.

74.   Do Calisthenics.   Initially start with a limited series of calisthenics each morning and night to not only keep your body fit, but establish muscle tone and work off some of your caloric intake. Exercise will also start to increase your normal metabolism. Your exercise regimen doesn't have to be exotic or lengthy. Start with 10 pushups, 10 sit-ups, 10 squat thrusts and 10 jumping jacks and you'll tone up, look better and feel better. If these numbers are too much for you, do whatever you can at first and slowly build up to those numbers until you find you can do them easily. That will indicate that your body has acclimated to that number of repetitions and has toned up so they come easily. Then, consider upping the numbers as you feel you can handle more. Of course, always check with your physician before starting any exercise program, regardless of how limited it is and always make sure to monitor your body's reaction whenever you exercise. You are always the one who is ultimately responsible for your well being, so if you have any reservations, make sure to honor them and check them out with your physician.

75.   Yoga.   You can join a yoga studio or do yoga at home with a video or one of the many health related television stations that display yoga classes regularly. Again, start out slowly and work your way up to more advanced yoga poses after you feel comfortable with the poses you're initially doing. You'll feel better for it physically and you'll burn off those calories more quickly and easily than you expected. Yoga will also keep your body toned and fit and you'll enjoy your new body and flexibility. It will also increase your body's metabolism which will, in turn, burn off any excess calories more easily. Try it, you'll like it.

One more important thought about exercise and your metabolism. It's been discovered that over **70%** of your metabolism comes from the normal functioning of body's organs. The rest of your metabolism is comprised of the effect of increased exercise. That means that the vast majority of your caloric burn-off is attributed to your normal activities - other than exercise.

The question then arises, "Is there a way to increase my normal metabolism in addition to exercise?" The answer is **yes**! There is a way of using Hypnosis to "turn up" your thermostat/metabolism so that it will burn off calories quicker than normal. You may want to consider seeing a qualified Certified Hypnotist to ask if they will assist you in directing the deepest part of your body/mind to "turn up the heat" so you can burn off calories even quicker - without harmful side effects that so many diet pills have to them.

At the same time, if you want to reinforce your will power to exercise you can also use Hypnosis to remind you to exercise and maintain your commitment to exercising regularly. Both issues can often be done within the same session.

WHAT TO DO ABOUT YOUR SWEET TOOTH

Many people have a soft spot for sweets. Its often called having a "sweet tooth." That's why there are so many bakeries, ice cream stores, candy stores and donut shops. Unfortunately, sweets are the downfall of most people. The worst part of eating sweets is they are generally made with refined sugar and pure fat (lard or things of that nature). You can be assured that sweets are not good for you or your body. They contribute to obesity, diabetes, ADD, ADHD, anxiety, stress, fear, worry and an assortment of other negative emotions. Don't those sound suspiciously like the same things that triggered you to smoke in the first place? You bet!

By eliminating sweets from your diet you will be taking yet another momentous step towards bringing about healing in your life and in your body. The question is how do you do it, right? Here are a number of suggestions to assist you. You won't regret using them and it's easier than you think.

76. Use EFT to Tap Away Your Desire for Sweets. To do it, focus all your attention on a cookie, cake or pie (or whatever sweet item you like most) and say these words while you tap on the side of your hand:

> "Even though I want this (choose one - cookie, cake, pie or other sweet dessert), Right Now, I love and accept myself anyway."
> "Even though I have to have something sweet at the end my dinner, I love and accept myself anyway."
>
> "I can't do without my sweets as a reward for getting through another day of stress, anxiety and worry, I love myself nonetheless."

Then tap all the meridian access points as outlined in the EFT chapter while saying reminder phrases such as "This cookie", "that cake", "that pie", "that ice cream," "this is my reward," etc. as you tap each meridian access point around the head and upper body. Watch how well it works to eliminate those negative feelings. It works wonders but you have to use the technique to make it work.

If you want to "super-charge" the technique, bring out a sweet item like a cookie or piece of cake, etc. and smell it and enjoy the smell as much as possible. Really get into the smell, look and feel of it. Then start tapping all the meridian access points as you continue to say things like "I really like that cake, pie, etc. and want to eat a piece of it right now."

As you continue to tap, you will begin to notice that the smell loses its good flavor and is replaced by a neutral or even a bad smell instead. Once the "good smell" has gone away, you'll usually find that any urge for that sweet item have gone away too and won't easily return.

77. Indulge yourself occasionally. Once in a while, have a sparse salad for lunch <u>and</u> dinner, and "save up" some calories for the day. Then trade in your "saved"calories for a nice dessert at dinner that has extra calories. You may find that it doesn't taste as good as you expected, but do it anyway just to acknowledge that you can do it. That way, you won't feel deprived and you'll notice how much your taste buds have changed and you may notice how you no longer crave sweet desserts as much as you did before.

78. Don't Keep Sweets Around. Avoid keeping sweets of any sort in the house and if you do buy them, limit what you buy to small sizes and limit your personal intake to just a few pieces a day. Monitor your weight to see how well you're doing with that approach. Most people find they not only avoid over-eating sweets that way, they learn how to control their cravings and often become proud of their accomplishment. Remember, "everything in moderation" is the way to in everything you do. In the alternative, you can also simply use EFT to eliminate any urge or craving to eat sweets.

79. Use Alternatives. If you and your family have established the habit of having a sweet dessert or treat every night after dinner or while watching TV, first try compromising by introducing low-fat ice cream, sherbert and/or fresh fruit instead of the normal sugary sweet dessert. You can also occasionally introduce just the fruit with a teaspoon of low fat whipped cream. It will make a big difference in the amount of calories and fat and will help you establish a new way of eating dessert in your family. That way, every member of the family can support each other and everyone will become thinner at the same time.

80. Schedule a Specific Period Without Any Sweets at All. Start with one day and then move up to two or three days or a week at a time. Then you can increase it from there. You may choose to use alternating days without sugar or other sweets. By doing this it gives you a goal and helps you to be more conscious and exercise more control in your eating habits. To accomplish this, do EFT on the issue of "I really want those sweets right now" and tap the negative urge away initially. It's amazing how those cravings will often vanish and stay away for weeks at a time with just a single tapping session, especially when you really want to eat them just before you start tapping.

It is also important to test your EFT results. After you've tapped on the sweets issue, you take out a piece of candy or other sweet that you enjoy and smell it and see how much of a drive to eat it is still in you. If the urges re-emerge, tap them away again until you're fully satisfied with your results and know they won't arise again. Don't let your urges control you - control them - using EFT.

81. Eat More Fresh Fruit. We know you've heard this before, but it really works. The fiber in fruit is very important to you for making whatever you eat last longer within your digestive tract. A person who eats enough fruit in their diet will automatically feel less like eating sweets. You'll also simultaneously add valuable enzymes to your system which will improve your digestion and elimination processes naturally. Fruit is very healthy for you and your body.

82. If You Absolutely Must Eat Sweets, At Least Be Smart about It! If you truly believe you can't do without your sweets, reserve about 100-150 calories per day for your favorite sweet to satisfy that urge. That amounts to about an ounce of dark or milk chocolate, half a slice of cake or pie, or about a 1/2 scoop of ice cream. Limit yourself to that amount and you'll usually be fine as long as you maintain your exercise regimen. Remember, you don't have to overdo it with the sweets to be satisfied. Eat just enough to feel satisfied and, after awhile, you'll notice that your taste buds will change and those same sweets won't hold the same allure as they did before.

83. Give your taste buds time to adapt. When you first start to cut back on sweets and substitute fruit, it may take a little time to adapt to the new tastes and textures. Give yourself a little time to adapt to the changes in your food plan and how you relate to them. Many of us have been brought up to think of sweets as a reward for being good as children and fruit as a necessity to eat, even though we did not necessarily like it. It's time to let that old thought pattern go and start seeing fruit as a new taste treat each time you bite into it. It may take a month or two to start looking forward to eating fruit, but give it time and you'll be rewarded for your patience. If you find you still have resistance to changing your perspective about fruit, use EFT on the issue and it will change quite quickly for you.

WHAT TO DO IF YOU ARE GAINING WEIGHT WHILE EATING HEALTHY

Sometimes people find that although they are watching what they eat, they still find themselves putting on weight and can't understand how or why. It's actually a simple equation. When you eat more calories than you're burning off, your body stores those excess calories for future use as fat. That's how you become fatter and gain weight. Therefore, you can either reduce your caloric intake or you can increase your metabolism. Doing both would be your best choice.

There are also a few other simple steps to keeping yourself slim and trim. Cut back on most fats, refined sugar and complex carbohydrates (starchy foods like bread and rolls, etc.) You will want to keep certain fats in your diet such as olive oil and fish oil, but otherwise, limit the amount of animal fat you include in your diet drastically.

You can also cut back on your intake of red meat since it contains a concentrated amount of calories in every ounce of it.

You can also follow a simple food combining regimen that keeps your protein (meat, poultry and fish) separate from complex carbohydrates (pasta, bread, rolls, etc.). The best part of the equation is you can mix vegetables with anything else or any combination of them. Just following that simple technique should be enough to keep you slim and trim.

That means you can eat meat, fish or fowl with vegetables - but no complex carbohydrates such as bread, pasta or potatoes. You can also eat all those complex carbohydrates with vegetables - but without any meat, fish or fowl. Notice that the vegetables are the central part of the equation which doesn't change. Just mix vegetables with pasta, etc. and keep away from adding meat, fish or fowl of any kind and you'll notice you start to shed the pounds.

Beyond that, here are some additional simple and practical suggestions that will help you eat more healthfully and maintain or reduce your weight as you continue to regain your health.

84. Read the Nutritional Facts Panel and Ingredients List. You may discover you've been eating more sugar, complex carbohydrates and preservatives than you want and never knew it. Also make sure to read on the package what the "serving size" is for each product. You may discover that what you thought was a serving (such as the contents of a particular drink) is actually more like two or three servings. It's also always best to eat foods that have the fewest ingredients. The fewer the number of ingredients, the better. Remember that the first ingredient is the largest ingredient. Make sure that things like sugar, salt, fats are placed last or close to last on the list. If there are any ingredients that you can't pronounce easily, they're probably not all that good for you and it would be best to steer clear of them.

85. Not All Smoothies or Energy Bars Are Low in Calories. Make sure to read the ingredients and calorie information as explained in the previous section and then act accordingly. You may want to pay special attention to the portion size of everything you eat. If the overall package says it contains two portions, that's a good indication you should only be eating half at a time. That way, if you eat something that is high in calories, you can still eat it - just eat less of it at one sitting. That way, you'll be able to enjoy it without taking in too many calories. In either event, the more you eat of anything, the more weight you'll gain, unless you work those calories off with exercise as explained earlier. There is just no getting around that simple fact, so accept it and work within that structure and you'll be successful.

86. Avoid Too Much Pasta. One normal serving of pasta is a dry cup of it, but many people often eat up to 4 cups at a sitting. Instead, choose one or two cups at most and eat it slower as you relish each bite. You'll soon notice the difference. If you want to reduce your weight, limit yourself to no more than one cup of pasta or eliminate it altogether for a few months and watch how your weight comes down. Otherwise, pasta can pack on the pounds.

87. Eat Protein and Vegetables. If you must eat pasta, always eat it separately from protein. Either eat meat, fish or poultry with a tomato sauce or eat your pasta with vegetables and sauce, but not the two types of foods together. When you keep the complex carbohydrates and the proteins separate, you'll usually notice a weight loss fairly quickly.

88. Eliminate Eating Bagels Completely. Especially eliminate eating the larger size bagels which have almost 500 calories each. Stay away from the butter, cream cheese and additional calorie rich toppings as well. Even what is known as a little "schmear" should be avoided. It all matters when it comes to calories. While they all add some taste to your bagel, they also add to your overall caloric intake at a tremendous level which you don't need or want in your diet.

89. Don't Skip Meals. By skipping meals, especially breakfast, you don't get your metabolism going which is helpful for burning off calories throughout the day. By the time evening rolls around, you will tend to eat heavier when your metabolism is already slowing down as your body readies itself for sleep. This often leaves your body heavier with the same amount of caloric intake. In fact, that's how sumo wrestlers put on so much weight and keep it on - by eating late at night and loading up on calories so their bodies don't burn them off while they sleep.

90. Eat Nuts Sparingly. While nuts are healthy for you, they are also filled with oils and are usually high in calories. That's one of the reasons why squirrels gather them in the Fall to carry them through the winter months. Eat nuts only as additional healthy snacks from time to time.

91. Don't Eat Out of the Container. Don't open the freezer and eat out of the ice cream container or open the cupboard and eat whatever comes into sight straight from the box. When you do that you can easily take in an additional 500-600 calories or more without realizing it. Instead, take out only a small serving, put it in a bowl or put it on a plate and put away the container. Padlock it if you must, but don't open that refrigerator/pantry door again for at least three hours and don't eat anything after 7 P.M.

YOUR BIGGEST PROBLEM - EATING LATE AT NIGHT

Late night snaking is the death knell to healthy eating. In fact, as mentioned earlier, it's actually the way in which Sumo Wrestlers pack on so much weight and then maintain it. They eat just before going to bed when their metabolism slows down dramatically during sleep. As a result, whatever you ate late at night remains in your digestive system throughout the night without burning it off due to your reduced metabolism as you sleep.

Here are some suggestions to change your late night eating habits. Follow them carefully and watch how successfully your weight loss and maintenance can be.

92. Eat Early and Regularly. We know you've heard this more than once before in this book but it's important enough to repeat. Eat breakfast early and make it your biggest meal of the day. Then eat lunch, and dinner at regular and reasonably appropriate times eating less at each subsequent meal. You'll be much less likely to overeat if your body is satisfied early in the morning and at each meal. Many people develop problems because they skip meals due to time constraints or stress at work, etc. and then try to make up for their lack of food during the day at night. That's exactly the opposite of the best way to lose weight.

93. Eat Early and Often. You can change the "three squares" a day into five or six smaller meals if that appeals to you. Again, always eat a big breakfast to get your metabolism up and running quickly as early as possible. That effectively sets the tone for the day and everything else you eat will be quickly metabolized too. Then eat "large snacks" or "small meals" every two hours until about 7 PM. After 7 PM don't eat anything else until the following day. While this may sound a bit extreme (and it is) it works and that's what this book is all about.

94. Eat at the Table. Eat your evening meal sitting down at the table. In fact, eat all your meals seated, focused and as still as possible. This will set the stage for honoring yourself whenever you're eating a meal instead of focusing on whatever is about to come next in your day or doing some other mental activity while you mindlessly eat. Take the time to be mindful of everything you do and you'll be far less likely to overeat.

95. Drink Cold Unsweetened Raspberry Tea. It tastes great without added sweeteners, keeps you hydrated and keeps your hands and mouth active. If you really need a little sweetness to go with the raspberry taste, add a little Stevia FOS to taste.

96. Drink Water. Drink a full glass of room temperature water whenever you feel hungry. It will dissipate your hunger right away and you'll be cleansing your body chemistry simultaneously.

97. Drink a Glass of Cold Water. While some may think this is a little controversial, you might consider drinking a glass of cold water whenever you feel hungry. The body will work harder to warm up the cold water and that burns off additional calories for about an hour afterward. It will also serve to hydrate and cleanse your body at the same time.

98. Change Your Nighttime Schedule. It may take a little effort, but it pays off big time. You need something that will occupy your mind and hands other than television which has a lot of food commercials on it which are purposely intended to make you hungry and get you to order their products. Switch channels whenever food or drink commercials come on instead of salivating over them. Then consider switching to reading, writing, games, the computer (Youtube.com, blogging, web surfing, etc.) or other hobbies that occupy you until you're tired and ready for bed. You'll find you will accomplish more and feel better about yourself than by falling asleep in front of the TV with an empty bag of chips in your lap.

99. Use EFT to Address Nighttime Emotional Eating. If you're eating at night because of negative emotions or self-limiting beliefs, use EFT to eliminate the emotional issues instead of eating to satisfy them. You'll feel better and eat less. Again, the way to do this is to acknowledge the negative emotions that are driving your nighttime eating binges. If it's loneliness, it might sound something like this:

> "Even though I feel so lonely at night that I just have to have some comfort food to make me feel better, I love and accept myself nonetheless."

> "Even though I get so lonely late at night when there's nobody to call and I'm all alone at home, that's when I reach for my sweets or those chips which I always regret the next day. Yet, I love and accept myself fully and completely anyway."

> "I feel so powerless to stop myself from reaching for my favorite comfort food when it's late at night and I'm all alone. Yet, I love and accept myself fully and completely anyway."

Change the wording to fit your own issues and use whatever wording that will best address your personal situation. As an example of how well this works, a client once called me the day after having an EFT session on this very issue and informed me that after the session she went to bed that night without food - for the first time in 30 years!

100. Closed at 7 PM. Post a sign on your refrigerator door that says exactly that and stick to it. This may sound funny at first, or even a little silly, but it works. Use it. If need be, put a lock on the refrigerator door after 7 PM. Whatever it takes to change your mind is fine, but you must take action to get it done.

101. Brush Your Teeth. It sends your mind a signal - "no more food for tonight. You've already brushed your teeth." If you find yourself getting ready to reach for some ice cream or something else after brushing, all you have to do is use EFT like this while looking at whatever it is you think you want:

> "I really want that ice cream..."
> "I can't stay away from that cake..."
> "Those chips would taste so good right now..."

Keep tapping all the meridian access points the entire time you're focusing on **wanting** to eat the sweets and salty stuff that's no good for you. By doing this, you don't even have to do the Set-Up or anything else. Just tap on the "snack" you want while you want it and the urge will go away quickly and stay away for a long time or perhaps even permanently. Of course, that distinction is made because sometimes there are other emotions driving your urge to eat them and it's a good idea to do more EFT tapping on that issue repeatedly whenever you're still feeling driven to eat it. That way, whatever negative emotion that underlies it will be addressed repeatedly and dissipated repeatedly, which often leads to a permanent cessation of the urge for that particular snack or food.

102. Sleep 7-8 Hours a Night and Start Early. By sleeping 7-8 hours each night, you will assure yourself of having the proper hormone levels which help your body naturally maintain its proper weight. An interesting study done at the University of Chicago found that when people were deprived of sleep, they exhibited lower levels of the hormones that control your appetite. Those who slept no more than 4 hours a night were more than 200% more prone to becoming overweight than those who slept at least 7 hours a night.

It's also important to go to sleep earlier than later. Remember that old saying, "Each hour of sleep before midnight is worth two after it," and in my personal experience, it is true. The best approach is to consciously set a bedtime and do your best to stick to it. If you really want to see something on late night TV, record it and watch it the next night during regular viewing hours. That way, not only will you save yourself from going to bed late at night, you'll also get to watch your favorite show while you're fully awake and better able to enjoy it.

103. Concentrate on Eating. Eat without doing something else at the same time. That means no TV, reading or sitting at the computer while you mindlessly munch away at food that you barely taste. By doing this you will help eliminate unconscious eating patterns which can be very deleterious to your health. When you eat, fully engage in it. Enjoy it. Close the book, turn off the TV and quietly pay rapt attention to whatever you're eating. Smell it and enjoy the smell. Taste it and savor the complexity of the tastes. Pay attention as you chew each bite until you finally swallow it.

Don't rush through your meal, washing everything down as you go faster and faster through your meal. Take the time to enjoy it and you'll find that there is more to enjoy than you ever realized. This is part of the overall process of becoming more Present with whatever you do. Eating is a prime example of how much more enjoyable it can be for you when you are Present with it.

POSITIVE AFFIRMATIONS TO
HELP YOU STICK TO YOUR NEW EATING HABIT

Many people like to have positive affirmations to reinforce these new positive thoughts and techniques. As an avid practitioner of EFT, I believe that all negative thoughts and self-limiting beliefs come from blockages within the meridian system. Once we eliminate the blockage, the negativity evaporates quickly and almost mysteriously.

As the negativity is eliminated, you are left with primarily positive thoughts and positive feelings. It's somewhat like blowing the clouds away that have been blocking the sun. Once they're gone the sun shines through. In reality, the Sun never went away. It was only blocked by the clouds. The same thing applies to us - once the blockages in your meridians are eliminated, the negative emotions are eliminated or "tapped away" and you are left with your normal positive feelings.

Nonetheless, for those who would feel better with the infusion of positive affirmations, here are a number of positive affirmations to serve just that purpose. They will also serve to fill in any "emotional voids" left while using EFT and after you've reduced any negativity down to zero. It can be helpful to offer the following positive affirmations in section 104 to the subconscious mind as you tap the various meridian access points at the same time.

104. Use EFT First. Before you start to use the "helpful phrases" which are also called positive affirmations, you should <u>first</u> use EFT to fully eliminate the negative phrases and self-limiting beliefs inside your mind and energy system. You can do this by tapping on whatever your craving or negative emotion is at the time it arises within you. Always phrase your words in the negative, such as:

> "Even though I can't do without my sweets*, I accept myself anyway." (Fill in *cake, pie, cookies, candy as it applies to you)

> "Even though I want that pie right now, I love and accept myself fully and completely."

> "I just love to eat my chips and dip while I watch TV now I feel like I'm being punished by not having them, yet I fully and completely accept myself nonetheless."

Remember you are going to tap on all the meridian access points after you've done the initial tapping on the Karate Chop spot of the non-dominant hand. As you tap each point, you should say a reminder phrase which is actually a part of the originating Set-Up phrase, such as:

> EB - "I really love my sweets."
> SE - "I just can't help myself."

UE - "I can't do without my sweets."
UN - "I really need to eat my sweets."
UM - "Why can't I just have one?"
CB - "I deserve a treat for being good."
UA - "I can't imagine doing without my sweets."
TH - "I really love my sweets."

Of course, modify the wording to fit your particular situation or issue and you'll usually find that the issue will start to dissipate quite quickly. Always continue with the tapping until the issue is completely eliminated and you're feeling no more urge for sweets or any other issue. That's when you can test it by putting a sweet item under your nose, sniffing it and seeing if you still have any urge left to eat it. If you do, then you still have more tapping to do on the issue. Its only over when you can smell the item and have no urge to eat it any longer.

105. Sample Positive Affirmations. After the craving is fully eliminated, you can then input choice words to the effect of:

"I choose to release my late night food cravings."

"I no longer need to eat late at night to find comfort."

"I choose to eliminate all my food cravings with EFT."

"I feel better without eating sweets."

"I notice my body is better off without those sweets."

"I choose to maintain my weight in a healthy fashion by eating healthy and nutritious foods."

"Everyday, in every way, I'm getting better and better at maintaining my new eating habits."

"I want to be around to see my children and grandchildren marry (graduate, etc.), so I'll do without (my cigarettes and) those sweets now."

"The smallest portion of sweets, carbs and meats are the best ones. The largest portions of vegetables are the best for me . . ."

"It's worse not being able to get into my clothes than being mindful of what I eat - as I eat."

"Even though I like my sweets, they don't like me."

"I choose to eat less and enjoy everything I eat more."

"I know I can do this. I know I can."

"I like being in control of my eating habits."

"I choose to remain in control of my eating."

"Life is a constant series of choices and I choose health."

"I know I can maintain my weight even though I've quit smoking."

"I like being a non-smoker for life who doesn't gain weight."

"I am a non-smoker who doesn't have to gain weight."

"I choose to remain a non-smoker who will never gain weight even though I've quit smoking."

WHEN EATING LESS ISN'T ENOUGH -
EXERCISE WILL DO THE TRICK

Oddly enough, most calories are used by the body during the normal metabolism process of the body's organs just going through their daily routine. In reality, exercise represents only about 20-30% of the body's caloric energy usage.

However, increasing and maintaining exercise does more than just burn up extra calories. It also helps increase muscle tone and is a means of natural stress reduction and builds the body's inherent ability to utilize food and air.

Exercise is an important component of a healthy lifestyle and should be done by everyone who quits smoking. It will rebuild the lungs as you exercise and move the blood through your arteries and veins and take away many of the blockages that have built up over the years of inactivity. In short, exercise is good for you and as a general rule you should do more of it. Of course, always consult with your physician before starting any new exercise program to make sure you're body and heart are up to it.

106. Overeating Does Not Happen <u>Because</u> of Exercise. This is a common myth that the more you vigorously exercise, the more you'll want to eat. Nonsense! That simply is not the case at all. Vigorous exercise won't make you want to eat more. In fact, it works exactly the opposite. When you exercise at any level of intensity or duration, it actually helps curb your appetite (and you feel better at the same time).

107. Always Keep Yourself Hydrated. When you're exercising, always make sure to drink lots of water. By the time you actually feel thirsty, you're more than likely already dehydrated. Instead, drink at least 16 ounces of water, sports drinks, or diluted fruit juices a couple of hours before you start to exercise. Then drink a glass of water an hour before and during your workout. Drink another two glasses after you finish. In other words, make sure you are fully hydrated at all stages of exercising.

108. Entertain Yourself While You Work Out. Consider taking an iPod along with you while you walk. That way you can listen to music, a book or a podcast which will keep you exercising longer and help you look forward to your next walk as well as the next podcast. Check the Internet or iTunes for a great selection of podcasts, many of which are free. Or, on the other hand, take nothing with you and be present with the birds, trees and sky and enjoy the entire experience for itself.

109. Yoga. Consider taking up yoga to burn more calories. You can burn 250 to 350 calories during a one hour class (that's about the same as you'd burn if you walked for an hour). Plus, you'll improve your muscle tone and strength, increase your flexibility, and enhance the endurance and stamina of your entire body. If you're disciplined, you can buy a yoga video and do it at home. If you don't know whether you will be disciplined, take one our of the library and see how well you do for a couple of weeks.

110. Drink More to Lose More. Drinking more water helps you to keep your weight down and cleanses your <u>lungs</u> at the same time. Otherwise, dehydration can set in and it will slow your metabolism down by 3 percent, or about 50 fewer calories burned a day. Over the course of a year, that could make a difference of losing as much as 5 pounds or more from your body. The key isn't how much you drink, but how <u>frequently</u> you drink it. Sipping small amounts regularly works better than drinking a full glass all at once. It's best to drink about 6-7 glasses of water a day. By keeping your body fully hydrated, everything works better and smoother including joints, digestion and elimination.

STOP EMOTIONAL EATING

We are basically emotional beings making emotional choices in our lives. It's only when the choice has been made that we then try to rationalize what we've done. Eating is a great example of how we are affected emotionally and how it can affect our body. When we eat due to emotional reasons, we aren't necessarily hungry. In fact, many people often eat to satisfy a different urge such as anxiety, fear, worry, boredom, seeking comfort or any number of other emotions. Many of these are the same urges that caused you to smoke in the first place and that's the primary reason so many people worry that once they stop smoking, they'll substitute eating for smoking and get fat as a result.

Emotional Freedom Technique (EFT) directly addresses and eliminates the negative emotional urges that cause so much aberrant behavior in people. To resolve emotional eating, it is best to use EFT when you are feeling the urge to eat without really being hungry. That's the best indicator you're about to eat because of your emotions rather than because you need food in your system. It's also the moment you can take matters in your own hands and tap that urge away. The simple fact that the aberrant urge arises within you is the very best reason to tap on the urge itself and watch as it dissipates while you tap. Make sure you completely eradicate the urge while you're feeling it and it's very likely it will never return.

Here are some additional techniques and suggestions that should help you find your way through emotional eating.

111. Take Control. By taking control of your emotional issues, you will ultimately change your eating habits. Many people eat because they're bored, tired, angry, anxious, nervous or want to satisfy some other urge, but don't feel like they can do it directly. So they use food as a substitute for love, affection, attention or any number of other feelings. As we explained in detail at the beginning of this book, you can use EFT to address whatever negative emotions are bothering you by eliminating the blockages in your meridians. Once you eliminate the blockages, those compelling negative feelings will dissipate quite quickly and you will notice how your eating habits change automatically because the driving forces behind them have been eliminated or resolved.

To accomplish this, first take a minute to recognize the negative emotions that are driving your over-eating. If it's a lack of love, for instance, all you need to do is acknowledge that feeling and do the

EFT tapping regimen using the following words. Here's an example of how it might sound:

> "Even though I feel so empty and lacking in love and affection that I want something to eat which will give me comfort, I accept myself nonetheless."

> "I just don't seem to have anyone in my life who loves me, so I usually turn to chocolate which makes me feel better for awhile - until I look at my scale or into my mirror - and then I'm horrified. Yet, I love and accept myself nonetheless."

> "I feel so lonely all the time that I feel like there's a hole in my soul that I have to fill with cookies and cake. Then I later regret what I've done and wind up hating myself for doing it. Yet, I accept myself just as I am regardless of what I've just done."

Of course, after you've done a Set-Up like any of the ones above, then you must do the tapping Sequence afterward in which you tap all of the meridian access points while saying Reminder Phrases like: "This loneliness", "This empty feeling", "I have to fill up this hole in my soul", etc. Continue to do the tapping on each feeling/issue you can identify until you fully resolve it. Once you've resolved enough issues, you'll begin to notice that your eating habits will start to automatically change and your weight will start to reduce naturally and easily.

112. Get Support. One of the best ways to maintain your weight is to join or form a support group or find a sponsor/friend. Try a smoker's support group and/or Overeaters Anonymous group. It is also suggested that you find a friend who is willing to use EFT with you, since it makes it easier to remember to use it and they will remind you to use it even when you forget. One other thing to remember is that EFT appears to work better when two people do it together rather than doing it alone. So when you do it with a friend, it will usually give you better results than if you do it alone.

When you "buddy up" with a friend, you'll find it's easier to stay on track and keep to your self-promises and goals than if you only have to answer to yourself. It also gives you someone to support your efforts when your will power gets a little weak and you just need a little emotional help.

113. Stress Can Be a Big Factor in Overeating. This is especially true for anyone who is already having difficulty with stress in their lives. Stress will almost always increase when you stop smoking if you've used it in the past to deal with stress. That's because when you've always relied upon smoking to lessen your stress and you now eliminate smoking, there's an automatic stressful response to your becoming a non-smoker.

Sometimes people who are under a great deal of stress will respond by eating more than usual so they have something to do with their hands and mouth. That's one of the greatest fears most smokers have before they quit. Again, you can use EFT to reduce whatever new stress arises and eliminate any new need to overeat in reaction to quitting. Here's an example of how to formulate the wording:

> "Even though I never thought it was going to be this hard to quit smoking, I love and accept myself nonetheless."

> "Ever since I quit smoking, all I seem to be able to think about is eating and now I'm considering going back to smoking just to stop eating. Yet, I love and accept myself anyway."

> "Once I quit smoking, I thought that was going to be all I had to contend with, but now I see that I have something else within me that is driving me to eat more than usual and I'm really concerned. Yet, I love and accept myself no matter what happens."

> "I thought smoking was my biggest problem, but now that I've stopped, I realize there were more unresolved emotions within me that are causing me

more problems than I ever expected. I sometimes feel powerless to change all this. Yet, I love and accept myself fully and completely nonetheless."

"I'm so afraid of getting fat just because I quit smoking that I'm thinking about going back to smoking again. Yet, I love and accept myself even if I go back to smoking."

"I can't ever go back to smoking because I'm so afraid of dying of lung cancer or something else. So now I feel like I'm trapped and I've lost my best friend - my cigarette. Yet I love and accept myself nonetheless and I'm doing the best I can."

114. Use "Computer Counselors" for Weight Loss. This is a "coach" of sorts that will help you over the computer or telephone to either maintain your weight or lose weight. Researchers put about a hundred people in an online weight loss program for a year. The ones who received weekly e-mails counseling them actually lost over 5 pounds more than those who received none. They were given weekly feedback on their diet and exercise regimens, had their questions answered, and given advice. Overall, it was a worthwhile experience. Best of all, they lost weight consistently.

Bonus: There is yet another benefit to reducing your caloric intake each day. There is a recent study from Johns-Hopkins University that demonstrates when you restrict your calories by approximately 30% your memory will actually improve. This applies to all ages and both genders, however, it primarily applies to those who already have a caloric intake above 2000 calories per day.

If you are already eating substantially more than 2000 calories a day, you can improve your memory by reducing that intake by about a third. It does not indicate that you should reduce your intake by a third if you are only eating about 1500-2000 calories a day. In those cases, it's better to change what you eat and add more fiber and leafy green vegetables to get the best use of your food with your body.

CHAPTER 4

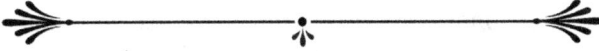

EMOTIONAL FREEDOM TECHNIQUE

Emotional Freedom Technique (EFT) is a simple tapping method which can result in profound and lasting effects on your physical and emotional well-being. The technique is simple so that anyone can learn it and effectively use it anywhere - any time.

Emotional Freedom Technique is on the cutting edge of alternative healing and medical treatments. This is because it combines both Eastern and Western healing philosophies into one powerful technique. It recognizes that beneath almost every physical problem lies an unresolved emotional issue which is exactly what Emotional Freedom Technique is intended to resolve. EFT works simultaneously on the mind and body by balancing the subtle energies of the body which are carried in the meridians. It can reduce or eliminate worry before undergoing medical procedures, eliminate phobias, reduce post-traumatic stress syndrome, reduce or eliminate chronic pain, stress and panic attacks, prepare witnesses to testify by reducing stress and fear, eliminate fear of public speaking and much more.

As most people know, we have different levels of our "mind" that do different jobs. There is the conscious mind, which is logical, rational and where our judgment, ego and will power are located. It figures things out and takes credit for the decisions we make. The subconscious mind is where our personality and emotions reside and where most of our decisions are actually made, regardless of how logical we think we are or how much we mull over a decision. We also have an unconscious mind which automatically runs our body so we don't have to consciously think about all the details of it.

Otherwise, can you imagine trying to remember to make your heart beat while you're in the middle of an argument or asleep? It wouldn't work too well, would it? That's why it's automatic.

Unresolved emotional issues often run our lives, whether we realize it or not. That's because we often react to situations which relate to earlier sensitized experiences in our lives without realizing it. For instance, if as a child, you felt abandoned by parents or loved ones (whether true or not), that feeling will often become a "trigger" throughout your life for certain behavior. As you reach maturity, anytime your experience even gets close to feeling like you're about to be abandoned, your subconscious will have you react quickly to avoid that same feeling from happening again.

Many times you may find yourself remaining distant or constantly moving from one relationship to another and thinking, "Why is this happening **to** me?" when, in reality, it's really your subconscious at work making sure you don't get hurt again like you did as a child. It hurt you too much then and the subconscious is not going to allow that to happen again. You may go through life getting only just so far in relationships before either ending them or putting up so many walls around yourself that the other person can't get close enough to "abandon" you. In effect, your subconscious "over-protects" you to the point of inadvertently hurting yourself because it doesn't know when to stop protecting you.

Keep in mind that the subconscious is not to be blamed for any of this. It is simply protecting you from being hurt again. Unfortunately, the subconscious usually doesn't know the full consequences of its protectionism. That's why the results of being protected can often lead to unexpected and, many times, unwanted results such as an inability to commit to relationships, addictions or weight problems, just to name a few.

When you encounter emotional, physical or chemical trauma, the energy meridians (pathways) that carry life-force energy (chi) become disrupted or blocked. That results in negative thoughts, self-limiting beliefs or pain. These may show themselves as fears, worry, sadness, grief or any number of negative emotions and/or negative reactions. Or they may show up as self-limiting beliefs like "I can't do anything right" or "Nobody will ever love me" or things like that.

We use EFT to open the blockages and bring the disrupted meridians into balance to neutralize the negative feelings and beliefs. As a result, you don't have to suffer the consequences of all those unresolved feelings any longer. We can already hear you thinking, "How am I you going to do that?" Well, it's actually a lot simpler than it sounds.

The basic premise is, *"All negative thoughts, self-limiting beliefs and pain come from a disruption in the body's energy system."*

That means that every time you have a negative thought or emotion, pain or a self-limiting belief, your meridian system has somehow been impacted by a physical, chemical or emotional trauma and became blocked. Now trauma sounds bad, like an auto accident, but it doesn't have to be that bad to impact upon your energy system. There are many levels of trauma and each of them has its own impact upon you depending upon how you perceive it. Remember, the subconscious doesn't make those distinctions logically. In fact, what might logically/consciously be thought of as a small matter may well be seen by the subconscious as a very significant experience. It's often confusing to us because our conscious mind judges our subconscious mind's actions without knowing how the subconscious mind functions. Our subconscious mind simply reacts emotionally to stimuli. On an emotional level, whatever the subconscious <u>feels</u> is how <u>we feel</u> about it.

What the conscious mind thinks needs to be addressed is not always the issue at all on the subconscious level. The subconscious level is ultimately where the healing work needs to be done. This is why EFT is so profound, because the conscious mind doesn't have to "figure out" the issue in order to do the work required to resolve your emotional issues. It is done on an energetic level.

MERIDIAN SYSTEM

Each of us has a meridian/energy system that runs throughout our body carrying life force energy. There are access points that allows us to access/affect the meridian by "tapping" on them. Tapping "breaks-up" the energy blockages within the meridian and resolves emotional and physical problems. We see the subconscious and unconscious levels of mind as integrally involved with the energy/meridian system.

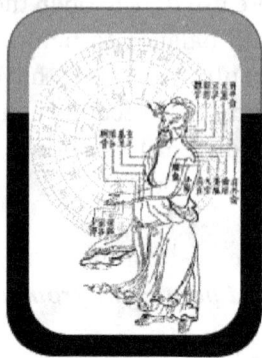

Ancient Chinese Meridian Chart

A good analogy of what we do with EFT is like tapping the top of a straw that has a little milk left in it. Once tapped, the blockage is broken and the milk flows out, leaving the tube open. The same thing happens when tapping the body's meridian access points. We tap the top of each meridian access point and break up the energy blockage within the meridian. This allows the body's energy to flow through that meridian again and changes your negative thoughts from negative to neutral ones again.

This is where the simplification comes in. In medicine, psychotherapy, counseling or other healing professions, to effect a change, one must first figure out what the problem is (diagnose it) and then specifically treat it. EFT does **neither** of these things. It simply acknowledges what emotion is being experienced in the moment and addresses it by tapping <u>all</u> of the energy meridians one by one. That way you can't miss the blocked meridian and relieve the blockage.

When the balancing of the body's energy meridians was originally developed in Tibet 5,000 years ago, the practitioner simply intuited where to place needles or tap. Then, as the treatment became more institutionalized the practitioner first had to diagnose the problem and then outline a specific treatment for it using meridian charts. That took precise needle placement or pressure to get results and the meridian access points could be at any of hundreds of points on the body. That system was primarily used for physical problems. With EFT, the number of access points used has been limited dramatically. By tapping multiple times, you almost guarantee that you will tap on the actual access points and get results. There are only 8 basic meridian access points to tap and perhaps as many as an additional 7 points in the more advanced form of EFT. The 8 basic points (1-8) will usually facilitate and accomplish all that is needed by most people.

DOING EFT

EFT is counterintuitive because it uses <u>negative</u> wordings to bring up all the negative feelings you have associated with the issue you are working on, whether you are conscious of them or not. This is a much deeper healing system than any cognitive/talk therapy because it does not rely upon any conscious analysis or thought. The healing is done on an energetic level within the body. By simultaneously tapping the access points and saying negative words, you are eliminating the blockage in the meridians that caused the negative feelings in the first place and you are left with neutral or positive feelings at the end of the process.

To do EFT, first focus on the negative issue, negative emotion or self-limiting belief and feel it fully. Determine how strongly you are feeling it on a scale of 1-10. This is called a SUDS (<u>Subjective</u> Understanding of Distress Scale). This is basically a "guestimate." Don't try to figure it out. Simply use the first number that comes to mind. Then, remember the number, since it will give you a reference point from which to start and will let you know how well you're doing as you use the technique. Now we'll turn to the actual technique and how it works.

THE SET-UP

The Set-Up sets the tone for the issue to be worked on and focuses your mind's attention on that issue. The Set-Up is also used to make sure you feel all the negative emotions associated with that issue to the fullest degree. That's how you get the best results. Many times, people object to saying any negative words to their subconscious mind, fearing that it may seize upon the negative thought and internalize it. That is <u>not</u> the case with EFT. In fact, by using the most negative words available, you will actually improve the result.

We do the Set-Up by tapping (with the first two fingers of your dominant hand) on the side of the opposite hand (the karate chop point - point 13 KC) continuously while saying, as an example, something like, *"Even though I have this anger within me, I deeply and completely love and accept myself."* By saying this, we are doing a couple of important things. First, we acknowledge that we are angry. Second, we tell the subconscious mind that, although it is angry (remember, emotions such as anger reside in the subconscious) the conscious mind (which is saying the words and judging the subconscious for being angry) "accepts" it and "loves" it.

Can you imagine the relief of the subconscious mind, which is only about 3-4 years of age on an emotional level, hearing that although it's being "bad" by being angry, it is accepted nonetheless by the "mature" conscious side of the mind?

That, in and of itself, is a very valuable and profound change of the relationship between the conscious and subconscious parts of the mind. Relief starts immediately.

Interestingly, some people can't say they love themselves, usually because they are their own harshest critic and don't love themselves - yet. If this happens, simply have them say, *"Even though I <u>don't</u> love myself, I accept myself nonetheless."* They can also say, *"Even though I can't say I love myself, I'm still OK,"* or **"I'm doing the best I can."** This will usually resolve the issue immediately as long as they continue tapping while saying those things.

THE SEQUENCE

After doing the Set-Up three times, we move on to the Sequence which consists of tapping the various meridian access points noted on the diagram at the end of this chapter. We also say part of the original Set-Up phraseology, such as *"this anger"* or *"I'm very angry,"* or *"I'm still angry,"* etc., either keeping the words the same or varying them slightly at each access point. This can be as simple as repeating *"this anger,"* or it can be as complex as allowing your mind to flow in a stream of consciousness about the anger issue. Either way, the system works superbly.

Remember, identifying the essence of the issue is important (that does not mean diagnosing the problem). The subconscious needs to know that you recognize exactly what the essence of the issue is before it will allow any resolution to occur. This is usually done with words, but it can also work by focusing on the emotion as you are intensely feeling it, even if you can't specifically identify it.

Sometimes an exact description of the issue will not be immediately obvious. In situations like this you can simply say, *"Even though I have this issue, I deeply and completely love and accept myself anyway."* Rest assured, the subconscious knows what the issue is and as long as you're feeling the feelings surrounding that issue, it will then be addressed within your energy system even if you can't find the right words to describe it. Intention is most important here. Focus on it. Feel it fully and then tap and you'll usually find success.

This also comes in handy when working with a new person who has a sensitive issue affecting them, such as rape, sexual abuse, etc. It may be so sensitive to them that they can't even speak about it openly, or bear to hear it spoken of by someone else. In such an instance, you can have them say, *"Even though I can't tell anyone about this, I accept myself fully and completely,"* or, *"Even though this issue is too sensitive for me to deal with, I accept myself fully and completely."* Change the words as needed and as you feel the issue arise within you. The subconscious will identify the issue easily because it's usually already obsessing over it. The person will usually experience a marked reduction in severity as long as they are focused on the issue and you tap on all the points.

Once you've finished the first round of the Sequence, stop tapping, take a deep breath, close your eyes and evaluate your level of discomfort about the issue you've just worked on. Determine between 1-10 where you are now and if it's less, but not yet a zero or a one, do the Sequence again. This time change the wording a little to the effect of, *"Even though I still have some remaining anger about this issue, I deeply and completely love and accept myself."* Then tap on all the points again, using Affirmations such as *"this remaining anger"* etc., until you finish all the points. Close your eyes and take a deep breath and determine where you are on the scale of 1-10. Continue the Sequence until you get down to a zero or a one. A one usually declines by itself to zero over time. A zero is when you can't find the issue in your mind any longer.

Sometimes your number may actually go UP after finishing a Sequence. This can be somewhat disconcerting to a newbie because you may become concerned that the technique actually made your condition worse. Relax. That's not the case!

What we have discovered is that when this happens, the reality is you actually completely eliminated the first issue quickly and your subconscious moved on to the next most important issue it has been holding onto automatically!

In order to verify this, close your eyes, take a deep breath and see if you can access the first issue - just as it was when you started. You will usually, if not always, find that you cannot access that issue at all. What has happened is that a different issue or a different aspect of the original issue has popped up unbeknownst to you and that's what you're now feeling.

That secondary issue can have a higher number than the original issue's number. Don't be frightened by such a turn of events! It is actually a very good thing because you have eliminated the first issue completely and thus opened up the subconscious enough to access the deeper issue that was hidden. You then have the opportunity to bring the true issue down to a zero and get the relief you ultimately wanted.

 If this should happen to you, use the closest words to describe the new issue, however if you cannot tell what the true nature of the new issue is, you may just say something to the effect of, *"Even though this new issue has come up, and I don't know exactly what it is, I deeply and completely love and accept myself anyway."*

You may then follow up with Affirmations such as *"this issue"* or *"this new issue"* etc. while doing the Sequence. Remember, the subconscious always knows what the issue is even if you can't consciously put words to it. It just usually works better with an accurate description. This sounds contradictory, and it is to some degree, but the right words just allow the technique to work better.

It is important to note that it is not necessary to tap very hard on each of the access points regardless of how high your SUDS level may be. The meridian access points will react to medium pressure. It is also not necessary to tap more than 5-7 times on each point, except the Nine Gamut point which is continuous. We recommend using two fingers to tap, because that way you can't miss the access points.

THE EYE LADDER

If you get the SUDS number down to a 3-4, there is a simple process that will eliminate the last of the charge. It's called the Eye Ladder.

Tap continuously with two fingers on the back of the opposite hand between the ring finger and the pinky, in the "valley" part of the hand, the Nine Gamut point (point 14). As you continue to tap, focus your eyes (without moving your head) down towards your feet as far as possible. Then, as if you were climbing a ladder with **five** rungs, move your eyes upward in five equal steps until your eyes are looking upward as far as possible without moving your head. Each time you move your eyes, repeat your affirmation such as "this anger" or "this remaining anger" or "all remaining anger." Continue this process until you are at a zero. That usually only takes one round of the Eye Ladder, but works best on a level 3-4 or less.

THE NINE GAMUT

The Nine Gamut is actually a synthesis of Neuro-Linguistic Programming and eye movement. In addition, the continuous tapping on the back of the hand balances the two sides of the mind, the conscious and the subconscious and gets them to work better together. It is a powerful adjunct to the primary Sequence when an issue won't budge.

To do the Nine Gamut technique, continuously tap on the back of the hand between the ring bone and the pinky bone, in the valley (point 14, Nine Gamut point), while doing the movements directed below.

Then, <u>without</u> moving the head, use your eyes to:
- Look straight forward for 5 taps
- Close your eyes for 5 taps
- Look straight forward again for 5 taps
- Look down and to the right for 5 taps
- Look down and to the left for 5 taps
- Move your eyes in a clockwise circle starting at 6 o'clock and return to 6 o'clock
- Reverse the movement starting at 6 o'clock and returning to 6 o'clock
- Count 1, 2, 3, 4, 5
- Sing or hum a tune (Happy Birthday works great)
- Count 1, 2, 3, 4, 5

While doing the circular movement, it is very helpful to have someone else move their fingers or hand in a clockwise and counterclockwise fashion so that your eyes can follow them. It gives your eyes something to focus on while moving. Ask them to watch your eyes closely.

If they notice that your eyes are "jumping," dancing or "skipping" parts of the circle, have them move their fingers back and forth across that section of the circle while you concentrate strongly on following the fingers in a smooth, flowing fashion. It has been our experience that when the eyes follow the circular movement smoothly over that spot, the issue being worked on often vanishes immediately or is reduced dramatically. As for counting to five, this is a rote memorization process and therefore, uses the left side/conscious mind. Singing a song uses the right side/subconscious mind. By alternating the two sides of the mind, you automatically re-balance the two sides of the brain so they will work together better.

THE APEX EFFECT

You may find that because EFT relieves you of your problems so quickly and effectively, your logical, conscious mind, cannot accept EFT as the reason for your relief. It may even attribute the most bizarre reasons for your success. You should know that EFT is often fast-acting and very effective and you should not be surprised if immediate success should happen to you.

At the same time, persistence is the best way to achieve the best overall results for your chronic conditions. Remember, EFT can be very effective - very quickly - most of the time. It may take some time to recognize just how profound EFT is at resolving your issues. If your usual negative feelings no longer arise and you are feeling more positive than usual, then that's a pretty good indicator of the shift.

To learn more about our regularly scheduled classes and groups, as well as more about EFT, Presence, hypnosis and the work that we do, visit our website at www.tedrobinson.com, www.hypno-eft.com or www.centerforinnerhealing.com. Same site, just three different ways of accessing it.

EFT ON A PAGE

THE PRIMARY STATEMENT
"The cause of all negative emotions is a disruption in the body's energy system."

EFT: A BRIEF EXPLANATION
Memorize The Basic Recipe. Use it on any emotional or physical problem by customizing it to your needs with an appropriate Setup affirmation and Reminder Phrase. Be persistent until all aspects of the problem have been resolved. Use it on everything!!

THE BASIC RECIPE- (Set a level of discomfort from 0-10 before starting)

1. The Setup...Repeat 3 times this affirmation:

Say *"Even though I have this anger, frustration, fear, etc., I deeply and completely accept myself."* while continuously tapping either the Karate Chop point on either hand (for specific issues) or rubbing one of the two Sore Spots (for intense and/or generalized issues).

2. The Sequence...Tap about 5-7 times with two fingers on each of the following energy points found on the attached diagram while repeating the Reminder Phrase at each point.

1	2	3	4	5	6	7	8	9	10	11	12	13
EB	SE	UE	UN	CH	CB	UA	TOH	TH	IF	MF	LF	KC

3. The 9 Gamut Procedure . . .Continuously tap on the Gamut point (9G) (14) while performing each of these 9 actions (the 9 Gamut is not used unless necessary):

(1) Eyes open (2) Eyes closed (3) Eyes open (4)Eyes hard down right (5) Eyes hard down left (6) Roll eyes in full circle (7) Roll eyes in circle in other direction (8) Count to 5 (9) Hum 2 seconds of a song (10) Count to 5. (Re-evaluate your discomfort level before continuing)

Stay Slim While You Quit Smoking

4. The Sequence (again)...Tap about 5-7 times on each of the following energy points while repeating the Reminder Phrase at each point.

Note: In subsequent rounds The Setup affirmation and the Reminder Phrase are adjusted to reflect that you are addressing *"this remaining"... (problem)* etc. (continue until at a zero).

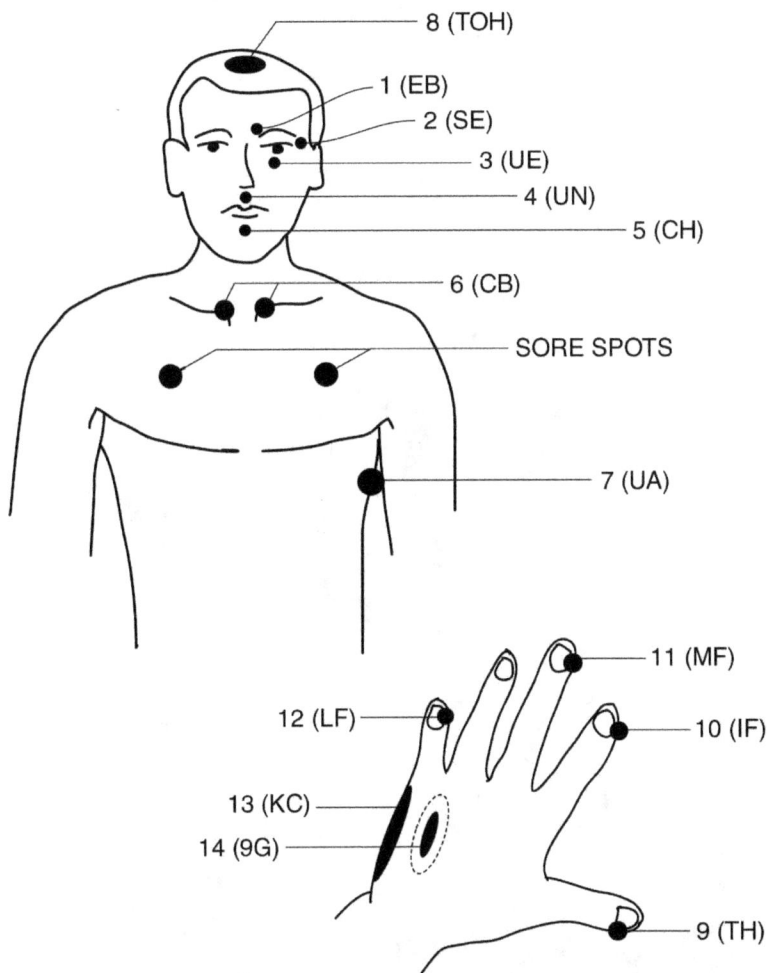

Stay Slim While You Quit Smoking

CHAPTER 5

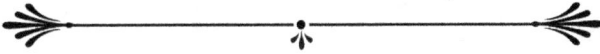

HEALTHY EATING SUGGESTIONS
AND RECIPES

THE HEALING POWER OF SOUP

Here's something that both scientists and grandmothers can agree upon. Soup has "magical healing powers" especially in the winter and it can help you lose weight at the same time. Soup is an ancient way of building immunity, warming you up and filling you up at the same time. A big kettle of soup can be easy to make and it can sit on the stove for hours and days and still be beneficial to those who partake. Soup should be a winter staple that nobody should do without. Here's a look at how soups can benefit you and heal your body and mind simultaneously.

An ancient Chinese proverb states that a good doctor uses food first, then, if that fails, he/she resorts to medicine. A healing soup can be your first step in maintaining your health and preventing illness. The therapeutic value of soup comes from the ease with which your body can assimilate the nutrients from the ingredients, which have been broken down by simmering over heat for a long time.

Soups can be very nutritious and they can flush out excess wastes from your body. Studies have found that people who eat just one serving of soup per day lose more weight than those who eat the same amount of calories, but without the soup.

Homemade soup is best for you because canned and concentrated soups tend to be crammed with salt and preservatives. Worst of all, they were made weeks or months ago and all the vitamins and minerals have been boiled away. It's best to make your own soup, using organic vegetables and filtered water whenever possible. That will eliminate the herbicides and pesticides that are often present in conventional produce which can play havoc with your immune system. When you make your own soup, you know exactly what went into it and you can rely upon the contents being fresh and organic if that's what you choose to use. Plus, you can use whatever spices you like best to get exactly the taste you want in your soup.

Immunity Building
Your immune system needs an array of minerals to properly function. The normal American diet rarely accomplished the task of providing you with all that your body needs. As you cook and slowly simmer soup, you gently release the minerals and nutrients in the ingredients you used and along with them, the energetic and therapeutic properties of the foods. Remember, cooking foods at high temperature, like rapidly boiling soup, destroys half the vitamins contained in the food so simmer your soup at a low temperature.

Soups to Improvement the Immune System
Start with a chicken or vegetable stock and bring it to a simmer at low heat - just enough to keep it hot, but not boiling. Then add any or all of the following immune boosting ingredients to taste and simmer at a low temperature for about 25-40 minutes: cut up squash, angle cut carrots, sliced cabbage, sliced fresh ginger, oregano, cinnamon, cayenne pepper, shallots, seaweed and/or shiitake mushrooms (if they are dried, soak them before adding). The reason there are no amounts given is because each soup made will be unique and different and it's a great way to experiment and make up new tastes.

Cabbage increases your body's immune system, helping it fight infection; seaweed helps cleanse the colon and ginger improves your digestion. Cayenne pepper will act to "burn out" any impurities in your body. It's better to have it hotter when it comes to pepper. Shiitake mushrooms contain vitamins and minerals that will help improve your immune system. All of the other ingredients will help your overall general health. It is suggested you eat this soup daily to effortlessly improve your immune system.

Detoxify Your Body
When you eat soup, you introduce more liquids into your body and that helps you flush toxins and waste from it. By adding various detoxifying ingredients, like those suggested here, you can double the detoxifying benefits to your body. These ingredients help to detoxify your liver. They also reduce your body's inflammation, increase blood circulation and help to improve your body's essential minerals to help achieve internal healing.

Soups to Help you Detoxify Your Body
Simmer the following ingredients (again, you may vary the measure of each ingredient according to your taste requirements) in a pot of water, vegetable or chicken broth over low heat: cabbage, collard greens, anise, Swiss chard, brussels sprouts, cilantro, dandelion, kale, fennel, mustard greens, garlic, watercress, leeks, cayenne pepper, shiitake mushrooms, daikon radish, fresh ginger, seaweed, turmeric and chili pepper. Drink 10 to 12 ounces 2-3 times per day. You can refrigerate any leftover and it will keep in the refrigerator for about a week.

Warm Yourself Up
Soups often provide both warmth and nutritious contents which the body craves, especially during cold weather. When you have soup, you are adding a lot of "warming energy" to the food. Warming foods that you will want to add to your soup can include: kale, leeks, broccoli, onions, spinach, turnips, garlic, yams, cayenne pepper, squash, shallots, scallions and parsley. When you use turmeric it helps improve your circulation which can be a great asset during colder weather.

Chicken Soup Really Does Work
Even if you never had a Jewish mother who made chicken soup, this is the opportunity for you to learn all about it and see its benefits. When you're sick, there is no better healing meal than soup. The

reason is because soup doesn't require much energy to digest, freeing your body to use its energy to fight off whatever is attacking you.

Chicken soup is the benchmark for all healing soups around the world and chicken and noodle soup is the mainstay of most homes. For good reason - it works! Studies have confirmed what mothers around the world have known for centuries. Chicken soup appears to relieve the common cold by reducing inflammation and helping to break up congestion with its rising vapors, increasing the flow of nasal secretions and clearing the nose quicker.

Even if it doesn't exactly cure the common cold, it will help relieve the symptoms and that helps in and of itself.

To make chicken/noodle soup, simply drop a whole chicken into a big pot of 2 quarts of water and add 1/2 cabbage, 2 sliced carrots, 1 onion and spices such as pepper to taste, 1/2 teaspoon parsley and simmer the entire pot for a few hours at low heat. Before long, the meat on the chicken will just fall off the bones (take them out) and you can then add your noodles and cook for a while longer to soften them. There you have it, Chicken soup with a smile.

BREAKFAST

Breakfast is the most important meal of the day. It is said that "You should eat breakfast like a king, lunch like a prince and dinner like a pauper." We learned this from our Grandfather who used to eat (no kidding) 2 scrambled eggs, a bowl of oatmeal, two pancakes and a couple of slices of toast every morning. He lived into his 80's and he never became overweight throughout his life. While that may only be one person's experience, it certainly is indicative of what can happen for anyone if they start each day with a big meal.

When you start the day with a big, healthy meal, it starts your metabolism up and gets it running at top speed early. That means the rest of the day your body is using up calories quicker than it will if you either fast at breakfast time or just eat a morsel or a cup of coffee. The faster your metabolism works, the thinner you remain or become and that's the purpose of following the suggestions in this book.

If you want to reduce your weight, then it's best to load up at breakfast time with a large meal that has few calories and lots of fiber. Fiber takes more energy for the body to digest and utilize and it takes more time to digest it. That means your food will last longer within your digestive system and that will provide you with a constant source of energy throughout a longer period of time and hold down your hunger.

Another approach is to drink a smoothie filled with protein which will fill you up and not add too many calories to your intake. See the entire line-up of smoothies starting at page 98.

EGG DISHES

Scrambled Eggs. Simple and easy to make for even the novice cook, scrambled eggs have it all. Simply break two eggs into a mixing bowl, whip with a whisk or a fork and a little milk. Then pour into a preheated frying pan with a little olive oil to prevent sticking. The eggs will cook very quickly once they hit the hot surface of the frying pan and you should not let them over-cook or they will get hard. Move the eggs around quickly with a spatula and cook to the consistency you like best. Some people like their eggs "runny." Others like them well done or in between. No matter how you like them, they are good for you.

Add some catsup or other ingredients to taste and you have a good start to your breakfast.

Omelettes. These are similar to scrambled eggs, but you add other ingredients to them and often turn them over onto themselves so they are self-enclosed. First start by whipping or mixing your eggs so they will be nice and fluffy. You may want to use a blender to get them really filled with air and make them fluffy. When you place them into a preheated frying pan, pour them all in at once (without moving them about, so they remain flat in your frying pan) and allow them to become just slightly cooked. (That means they'll be solid enough to hold together if you wanted to flip them over, but not hard or fully solid.) Then add whatever ingredients you want into them, fold them over onto the lower half and you have an omelette.

Some great options are a **Spanish Omelette** which basically has onions, peppers, ham and whatever hot spices or hot sauce you can stand into the mix and you actually blend all the ingredients together with the eggs before you place them into the frying pan.

If you want a simple **Swiss cheese omelette** or a **mozzarella omelette** you may add the cheese in on top of the eggs and then fold it over onto itself and cook until it's the consistency you desire.

Of course, you can add any combination or types of vegetables, such as broccoli, mushrooms, sweet potato or regular potato slices and a host of any other type of vegetable you want to any omelette as long as they are slightly cooked before you start your eggs so they are all fully cooked at the end for serving.

Oatmeal. There are a number of different types of oatmeal available, however, if time is an issue for you in the morning, then buy quick cooking oatmeal and it only takes a minute to cook or you can simply add hot water to a packet of oatmeal and stir it up.

When it comes to serving oatmeal, simply place it in a breakfast bowl and add some skim milk, almond milk or soy milk. If you want to sweeten it, you may use brown sugar, natural maple syrup or any of the artificial sweeteners you like. It becomes a really enjoyable dish if you add slices of apples, peaches, blueberries or other berries.

Cream of Wheat. This is another breakfast cereal that goes back a long time and you can buy in your grocery store. It is easy to make and only takes a few minutes of boiling on your stove to finish.

Serve in a breakfast bowl with a little almond milk, soy milk or skim milk and add the sweetener of your choice and your just about done. Add some fruit and/or berries and you'll have a nice meal to start your day.

Hot Pockets, Breakfast Bars and Other Processed Food. These are not suggested products to use for your breakfast meal. While they are very convenient, they are also processed to the point that they have very little nutritional value and usually have lots of sugar and preservatives in them. Both things to be avoided.

Pancakes. While these are usually very high in complex carbohydrates, butter and sugar, there are ways to make pancakes that are more nutritious and lower in fat and calories. Here is one suggestion:

Whole Wheat Blueberry Pancakes (With Applesauce)
 Ingredients:
  1 cup sifted whole wheat (unbleached) flour
  3 tablespoon of natural unsweetened applesauce
  1 egg, lightly beaten
  1/4 teaspoon salt
  1/4 teaspoon vanilla extract
  2 teaspoons baking powder
  1 teaspoon butter or butter substitute (melted) or olive oil
  1/4 cup skim milk
  1/2 cup of blueberries (thawed if frozen or washed)

Melt butter in a small pot and set aside. Mix together the flour, applesauce, egg, salt, vanilla extract, baking powder, melted butter or olive oil and skim milk until smooth. Heat skillet or grilling pan until a drop of water "dances" on the surface. Lightly oil or spray with Pam and pour your pancakes out one by one to approximately 4" in diameter. Drop a number of blueberries into each pancake as it starts to cook and when you see bubbles coming up through the top it is time to turn them over. They should be golden brown on both sides to be completely cooked in the middle.

You may add additional blueberries to the top of your pancakes and natural maple syrup is suggested since it is basically organic and you won't need much.

ALL SMOOTHIES ARE NOT THE SAME - BUT . . . THESE ARE GREAT!!

A smoothie can be just the thing to tide you over when you have to eat something sweet but don't want to eat too much. They are also great for breakfast and TV snacks instead of high calorie chips and dips.

Almond Delight. Here's a great idea for an Almond Smoothie that is low in calories, satisfying to drink and will be great for breakfast or at snack time.

> **Ingredients:**
> 1 cup low fat unsweetened vanilla almond milk
> 3/4 cup frozen low fat vanilla yogurt
> 1/4 cup roasted almonds
> 6 oz. low fat firm tofu or protein powder equivalent
> Optional - add 1/2 teaspoon of vanilla extract or to taste

Mix all ingredients in a blender and blend to the consistency you like best. Add ice if you want it cold. This makes two glasses or half the ingredients to make one glass. Make sure to blend at high speed to assure that all nuts are cut into small pieces.

Green Monster Drink. This is a great way to get all your greens in one drink.

> **Ingredients:**
> 1 heaping tablespoon green powder of your choice
> 1 cup cold fruit juice or water
> 1/2 cup frozen berries
> Optional - 1/2 cup ice and berry preserves for sweetness or add Stevia

Powdered greens will help you get through the day with plenty of energy and keep your blood sugar consistently high throughout the day. Use any green powder you want. They are usually sold at health food stores. We've used Greens+ and Nutrigreens successfully.

Asparagus "Alternative" Drink. This is a good alternative to the Green Monster Drink, however, it still incorporates lots of greens in it and may actually have additional healing value to you. All you do is take fresh, canned and/or frozen asparagus in whatever amount you wish to drink and place it in your blender. Turn your blender to "Puree" and let it blast its way through every last bit of that asparagus until you have nothing left but thick juice. You may add a little green powder to cut the singular taste of asparagus a bit or you may choose to add some sweetener to make it a little more palatable, but make sure to dilute it before drinking so it is easy to swallow. This drink will add great anti-oxidative quality to your drink and will start or continue the process of de-acidification within your body.

"Anti-Cancer" Shake. While this may not have yet been proven to affect cancer one way or the other, it certainly can't hurt to use it as another great shake to start your day or as a snack anytime. The ingredients in this recipe contain anthocyanins, may help in the cure of colon and breast cancer and more.

Ingredients:
1 1/2 cups of low fat milk, almond milk, rice or soy milk
1 medium sized ripe banana (sliced and frozen)
1/4 cup fresh or frozen blueberries
1/4 cup fresh or frozen raspberries (unsweetened)
1/2 teaspoon vanilla extract
1/4 teaspoon almond extract
A pinch of cinnamon
A pinch of Stevia FOS if needed - to taste

Combine all the ingredients in a blender and stir until you get the consistency you like most.

Bananadana Smoothie. This is a great way to get some needed niacin into your diet and have a nutritious, energetic and tasty treat at the same time.

Ingredients:
1 banana
1/2 scoop protein powder
1 cup low fat almond milk
1/2 cup ice
1 teaspoon vanilla extract
Add Stevia to taste

Mix all ingredients in a blender for about a minute to your taste and consistency.

Frozen Fruit Surprise Smoothie. This is a great way to use up all of your left over fruit that was about to go bad when you remembered to freeze it for another day. Well, this is that day.

Simply place 3/4 cup of frozen vanilla yogurt and add whatever frozen fruit you have on hand and a cup of ice. Blend them together until they are the consistency you like. Add enough Stevia, honey or maple syrup to make it sweet enough for your taste and enjoy. The ingredients will vary each day/week according to what you've kept frozen. That's the surprise!

Peanut Butter Smoothie. For those who like peanut butter and but don't want to add on the calories, here's the one for you. If you find it is too thick for your taste, simply add some ice and blend at high speed.

Ingredients:
1 1/2 scoop protein powder of your choice
2/3 cup frozen vanilla yogurt
1/2 cup almond milk
2 tablespoon natural peanut butter
add Stevia sweetener to taste

Strawberry Sunrise. This is a great way to start the day since it will provide you with a nutritious drink and give you your first helping of fruit of the day. Makes a little more than a full glass of drink.

Ingredients:
2/3 cup frozen vanilla yogurt
1/2 cup vanilla unsweetened almond milk
1 tablespoon strawberry preserves
1/2 cup frozen strawberries
Optional - add some additional crushed pineapple to taste for a surprisingly pleasant taste treat

"Muscle-Bound" Protein Drink. This is one of the best ways to enjoy a great protein drink. Mix all the ingredients below in a blender and enjoy it, knowing it's high in protein and minimal in fat.

Ingredients:
1 scoop protein powder
1 cup frozen vanilla yogurt
1/2 teaspoon vanilla extract
1/2 cup ice cubes

SALADS

This is perhaps the best way to reduce or maintain your weight and still not feel deprived or low on sugar later. Salad provides lots of roughage to help you feel full longer and won't leave you feeling flat before the next meal.

Here are two low calorie dressings that can be added to just about any type of foundational lettuce or other salad components you wish. Remember, the more diverse the components in a salad, the better it is:

Balsamic Vinaigrette Dressing

Ingredients:
3/4 cup extra virgin olive oil
1/4 cup balsamic vinegar
1 tablespoon oregano
1 teaspoon minced or crushed and diced garlic
Sea salt and fresh ground pepper to taste

Simply blend the above ingredients in a bowl and mix. Add salt and pepper to taste. Makes approximately 1 cup which will serve 4.

Lemon-Ginger Salad Dressing. This is a great dressing that will add a zest and spicy quality to any salad you put together.

Ingredients:
3 tablespoons fresh lemon juice
3 tablespoons fresh water (filtered preferred)
2 tablespoons olive oil
2 teaspoons pectin
1/2 small garlic clove, diced
1/4 teaspoon crushed crystalized ginger
1/8 teaspoon ground ginger
1/8 teaspoon ground cumin
pinch of salt
pinch of pepper

Pour ingredients (except for crystalized ginger) into a processor or puree in blender until it reaches a medium thick consistency and then add crystalized ginger afterward. Refrigerate before using. It will last as long as 3-4 days if refrigerated. Great over any salad.

Shrimp and Mushroom Salad (with Orange Dressing). This is a great tasting and highly beneficial salad that serves 4. The Orange/Ginger dressing adds a tangy and sweet taste.

Ingredients:
2 dozen large shrimp, de-veined, cleaned and cooked
1 cup shiitake mushrooms sliced to 1/4"
1 medium sliced green or red pepper
2 cloves of garlic
2 teaspoon chopped ginger
1 pound container of your choice of salad greens
1/2 pound snow peas (cleaned and de-strung)
1/2 cup of olive oil (extra virgin)
1/2 cup thin sliced Vidalia onion
2 teaspoon rice vinegar
2 teaspoon soy sauce
1 tablespoon Thai sweet-hot chili sauce
1 teaspoon chopped cilantro
1 orange, zested (skin of orange skin) and squeezed

Heat olive oil in saucepan or Wok at high heat and add garlic and ginger until slightly browned (less than a half minute). Add the mushrooms, onions, snow peas and sliced peppers, stirring constantly for about 3-4 minutes. Add the shrimp and continue to stir until the shrimp turn slightly pink. Add the orange juice and orange zest and remove from heat. Stir in the rest of the olive oil, soy sauce, chili sauce and cilantro and mix the entire contents fully. Serve over the mescaline and spread the dressing over the entire salad or offer to place it in individual pouring bowls next to each guest.

Asparagus, Turkey and Whole Wheat Pasta Salad. This is a great protein-enhanced salad that also adds the freshness of spring asparagus and Vidalia onions together with fresh quartered lemon. A great taste with few calories. Serves 4.

Ingredients:
6 fresh asparagus stalks or 3/4 cup of frozen asparagus
6 oz. Cooked fresh turkey, diced
4 oz. of whole wheat pasta of your choice
1/4 cup chopped Vidalia onion
4 leaves of leaf lettuce of your choice
2 tablespoons of blue cheese (crumbled)

Cook pasta until tender, drain and rinse in cold water to cool it off. Cut asparagus stalks into 1" pieces and steam until soft, but still crunchy. Drain on paper towels. Break up lettuce into bite sized pieces and place in mixing bowl and add pasta, asparagus, onion and turkey and toss thoroughly. Refrigerate until ready to serve. This salad will usually last up to three days if properly refrigerated.

You may wish to use the lemon slices alone as dressing or you may choose any low calorie dressing you wish.

Tuna Salad. Here's a quick way to make a high protein salad that is tasty and low in calories at the same time. Simply buy canned whole white tuna in fresh water, not oil, and mix with a tablespoon of low calorie mayonnaise. Add some diced celery, onions and carrots and you have some great tuna salad.

If you want to make your tuna salad even lower in calories and fat content, substitute mustard, either brown or yellow, for the mayonnaise and you'll have a spicier taste and far few calories and fat content.

Last, but not least, if you want to really cut down on the calories, simply eat drained tuna without any condiments whatsoever.

Seared Tuna Salad. This is a great dish for those who like their tuna nearly raw, similar to sushi, but with a "little heat" on the outside to sear the taste in. Simply take whatever size tuna steaks you wish to use, usually less than 1/8 pound per person and place them on a grill, either interior or exterior type, using medium high heat. Only allow them to sit on the grill for a few minutes - no more than 3-4 minutes. That way, the tuna will become slightly grey on the outside and the inside will stay red and raw.

Remove them from the grill and slice them in 1/4" strips and then cut them in no more than 1" sections and serve over your favorite salad.

Perhaps the nicest salad to use in this situation is a spring salad mix that you can buy at any grocery store and use a half a lemon as the basic salad dressing. You may wish to add any other low calorie salad dressing for a bit of flavor or a small amount of soy sauce and a little light green wasabi paste to add to the spicy flavor of the dish without adding calories.

Apple Walnut Salad. Fresh fruit adds refreshing zest and flavor to a tossed salad. Nuts top off the nutrition and adds crunchy interest. Serves 4.

Ingredients:
2 cups of shredded lettuce of your choice
4 large red-leaf lettuce leaves
1 medium sized apple (Fuji or Delicious)
1 celery stalk sliced and diced

Dressing:
6 walnut halves - chopped
3 tablespoons apple juice, unsweetened
1 tablespoon apple cider vinegar
1 tablespoon vegetable oil or olive oil
1/8 teaspoon paprika
1/8 teaspoon salt

For the dressing, combine all dressing ingredients in a container with a tight fitting lid and shake vigorously.

Core the apple and slice. Add the apple pieces to the chopped celery and shredded lettuce and toss in a salad bowl. To serve, equally divide the mixture into four sections and spoon them onto the red-leaf lettuce leaves. Serve with the Walnut dressing

Spicy Tomato, Pepper, Cucumber, Mint, and Parsley Salad. This is a great Middle Eastern salad and dressing which is intended to stand alone as a salad or it can be with grilled meat, fish and fowl.

Ingredients:
Salad:
4 medium ripe fresh red tomatoes (plum are sweetest) diced
3/4 cucumber, sliced and diced
1/2 cup coarsely chopped arugula
3 scallions (include the green), thinly angle sliced
1 cup coarsely chopped fresh flat-leaf parsley
4 tablespoon chopped fresh mint
1 1/2 tablespoon chopped fresh thyme
3 jalapeño peppers, seeded and diced
2 1/2 tablespoon capers, rinsed and drained

Dressing:
4 tablespoon virgin olive oil
1 1/2 tablespoon lemon juice
1 1/2 tablespoon balsamic vinegar
2 teaspoon grated lemon zest (sliced skin)
Sea salt and freshly ground black pepper to taste

Cut the tomatoes in half and remove the seeds. Dice the tomatoes and drain them in a strainer. Add tomatoes to the cucumbers, greens, scallions, herbs, jalapeños, and capers in a salad bowl.

For the dressing, mix the olive oil, vinegar, lemon juice and lemon zest. Add salt and pepper to taste. Add to the salad and toss. Add additional seasoning to taste. Refrigerate before serving.

LUNCH AND DINNER ENTRÉES

When it comes to making meals, less is more when you want to maintain or lose weight. That doesn't necessarily mean you have to eat less, you just need to learn to eat right. However, when all else fails, then it is time to simply learn to eat less and enjoy it more.

The primary reason lunch and dinner meals have been included in the same section is because of the old adage "Eat breakfast like a King, lunch like a Prince and dinner like a pauper." In this instance, you may eat any of these entrees either for lunch or dinner, but you may want to reverse the manner in which you used to eat and eat your larger meal at lunch rather than dinner.

Here are a few recipe suggestions on how to maintain your weight while enjoying hearty meals.

POULTRY

Whole Chicken. Simply take a whole chicken and pop it into a "chicken grill" put out by George Foreman and grill it upright while the grease comes out the bottom. It usually takes about 25-45 minutes to completely grill it. It stays moist due to the short time in the grill and it gets browned simultaneously.

Serve with mashed cauliflower and frozen peas and you have an excellent and timely meal that is low in calories and high in nutrition.

Mint and Garlic Chicken. This is a great summer dish, especially if you have plenty of fresh mint and/or garlic. It is light and low in calories and goes well with green vegetables and sweet potatoes. This recipe is for 4 people:

Ingredients:
4 boneless breasts - skinned
1 tablespoon fresh lemon juice
1 tablespoon olive oil
1 tablespoon low sodium soy sauce
1 teaspoon chili powder
1/2 cup fresh mint leaves
4 fresh cloves of garlic
1/2 teaspoon fresh black pepper

Blend the lemon juice, olive oil, soy sauce, cleaned garlic, mint leaves, chili powder and black pepper in a blender until it is finely chopped and fully mixed. Marinate the chicken breasts in the refrigerator for a minimum of 3 hours.

Grill for approximately 10-15 minutes, basting with the marinade to keep the chicken moist. You can also saute the chicken in olive oil until cooked.

Serve over brown rice or couscous and add a serving of broccoli for greenery. Add some fresh mint leaves to the top of the chicken for further garnish and add a section of fresh lemon to add some zest.

Mediterranean Wrap. This wrap is stuffed with chicken tenders or small sections of chicken, couscous with a hit of lemon and a healthy dose of fresh herbs. Serves 4.

Ingredients:
1/2 cup water
1/3 cup couscous, preferably whole-wheat
1 cup chopped fresh parsley
1/2 cup chopped fresh mint
1/4 cup lemon juice
3 tablespoons extra-virgin olive oil
2 teaspoons minced garlic
1/4 teaspoon salt, divided
1/4 teaspoon freshly ground pepper
1 pound chicken tenders or small sections of chicken
1 medium tomato, chopped
1 cup chopped cucumber
4 10-inch spinach or sun-dried tomato wraps

Follow directions for cooking the couscous. Fluff with a fork and set aside. Meanwhile, make the dressing by combining the parsley, mint, lemon juice, oil, garlic, 1/8 teaspoon salt and pepper in a small bowl. Set dressing aside.

Stay Slim While You Quit Smoking

Toss chicken in a medium bowl with 1 tablespoon of the dressing and the remaining 1/8 teaspoon salt. Place the chicken in a large nonstick skillet and cook over medium heat until cooked though, 3 to 5 minutes per side. Transfer to a clean cutting board. Cut into bite-size pieces when cool enough to handle.

Stir the remaining dressing into the couscous along with tomato and cucumber. To assemble wraps, spread about 3/4 cup of the couscous mixture onto each wrap. Divide the chicken among the wraps. Roll the wraps up like a burrito, tucking in the sides to hold the ingredients in. Serve cut in half.

Lemon Chicken. This is a wonderful dish that not only tastes great, but is also high in protein.

> **Ingredients:**
> 4 chicken breasts (deboned)
> 1 1/2 tablespoon olive oil
> 1 whole lemon
> 1 teaspoon oregano
> 1/2 teaspoon fresh basil, chopped

Heat the olive oil in a frying pan until hot. Coat the chicken breasts with the oregano and basil and saute until fully cooked. Just before taking the chicken out of the pan, cut a lemon in half and squeeze over the chicken breasts. Squeeze the other half over the chicken breasts just before serving.

Lemon Chicken with Artichoke Hearts. Use the same recipe above but add the artichoke hearts with the lemon once the chicken is cooked and stir for an additional 7-9 minutes.

Roasted Turkey. That's right. Just like at Thanksgiving - only every other week or so. Turkey makes a great meal any time of year, it's low in fat content and low in calories. It also makes great "left over" sandwiches, especially if you add some cranberry sauce to them. Or try them with mustard or low fat salad dressing instead of mayonnaise to reduce fat and cholesterol.

Cook a 10-15 pound turkey in a 350 degree oven for about 2 hours or until fully cooked (most have those little pop-up thermometers on them today that tell you when the turkey is fully cooked inside).

Baste the turkey as it is cooking every 15-25 minutes, making certain that it doesn't dry out or for even better results, cook it in an oven baking bag to keep it moist. You can find baking bags in most food stores.

Barbequed Turkey. This is a recent addition to ways to cook turkey and many people who love to BBQ especially enjoy it. They often mention that you can change the taste of the turkey by changing the type of wood you use in your BBQ instead of just using gas. Quite simply, place your turkey on a spit if you can and keep basting it as you continue it on medium to high heat. Or, if you can't fit it on a spit or you have none, keep turning it as you cook it so it gets done evenly throughout. Some people simply sit it up on its rear end and prop it in place and then baste it from the top. Depending upon the size of the bird, it will usually take between 11/2 - 2 1/2 hours to fully cook. Of course, since this will depend upon a number of variables, check to see that the entire bird is cooked before serving by cutting deeply into the breast and making certain that it is white throughout.

PORK

Pork Chops with Orange Slices. This is a great dish that adds a little citrus flavoring to the taste of pork chops. Serves 4.

> **Ingredients**:
> 4 pork chops
> 2 oranges (sliced)
> 1 ½ lb yams or potatoes

1 avocado
1 Tablespoon chopped parsley
2 Tablespoon olive oil

First brush on the olive oil onto the chops and grill them for approximately 5-6 minutes, depending upon thickness. Make certain that they are cooked throughout by slicing and checking for doneness. Next, take the sliced oranges and place them on the grill for a short time just to get the color of the grilling marks on them and to soften them up a bit.

Prepare the yams or potatoes by pealing and slicing them in 1/4" sections and you may either place on the grill and cook them until they are soft and cooked or you may place them in a skillet with olive oil until they are fully browned and thoroughly cooked. Set aside in a warming tray or bowl.

Scoop out the avocado and mix it with the chopped parsley and a little bit of orange to taste. Thoroughly mix and serve in a separate bowl for addition to the meat. Serve entire meal on a serving plate with the orange slices acting as garnish for the pork chops and the avocado mixture and yams or potatoes as a secondary dish.

If the orange slices are not sweet enough for your taste, you may always substitute or add canned Mandarin Orange slices to taste.

BEEF

While most books about weight control acknowledge that eating red meat of any nature is no longer an acceptable way to lose weight, these recipes are included for those who want to eat beef from time to time and still keep off the pounds.

Hamburger. This is America's favorite backyard barbeque meal. Usually, it is simply chopped beef that's been formed into "patties" and thrown on the BBQ until browned. However, here's a way in which you can add some additional ingredients and make your hamburgers a little more tasty and a little less beefy.

Simply add a tablespoon of breadcrumbs and spices such as oregano, cumin and paprika to each raw hamburger as you're forming them in your hands and knead them into the mixture until they are fully formed. These added ingredients will add some spice and substance and will make them even better than before.

Flank Steak. Choose a medium fatty flank steak at your grocery, making sure there are some small white veins in the meat so that it will stay moist as it is being cooked. Place under the broiler of your stove and broil for 10-12 minutes depending upon its size and depth. Make sure to turn it over from time to time so that it gets done on both sides. Check whether it is done from time to time by cutting into the middle of it to see if it is still red/pink inside. Cook to your own preference.

Roasts. The easiest thing to prepare since all you need do is place it on a roasting pan and pop it into your oven at 350 degrees and leave it there until it is done. How long you specifically leave it depends upon how well done you want it to be.

If you want your roast to be an even easier dish, simply cut up potatoes, onions, peppers, carrots and any other vegetables you want to eat with it and place them around the roast about 6-10 minutes before taking it out of the oven. That way, the vegetables will cook quickly around the roast and it will make a great side dish. Don't include peas in the mix since they will cook much faster than anything else. Simply cook them separately and add them to the table when they are done.

London Broil. This dish is a favorite of most meat eaters who love their steak. Purchase an extra thick (about 1 1/2") steak or top round cut of steak in whatever size you require for your family. Serves 6.

Ingredients:
1 1/2" thick London broil, about 1 1/2 pounds
2 tablespoons olive oil
1 tablespoon diced onion
1 garlic clove, chopped
1/2 cup red wine
1/2 teaspoon pepper
1/4 teaspoon salt
1/4 teaspoon oregano
1/4 teaspoon basil
1 bay leaf

Trim fat from steak. Combine all other ingredients in a container and marinate beef for at least a 6 hours, turning regularly until. Preheat your broiler or grill and place your marinated London broil under or on the heat and cook. Do not allow the steak to become overcooked or it could become tough and chewy. Using a sharp cutting knife, cut on a 45 degree angle and serve.

SEAFOOD

Pan Seared Pepper Encrusted Tuna Salad. This is a great way to eat tuna and a salad at the same time and dramatically save on calories. It's also very simple to prepare. Serves 2.

Ingredients:
6 ounces of fresh tuna steak
fresh ground pepper, to taste
2 peeled and sliced avocado
2-4 tablespoon of dried cranberries
low sodium soy sauce, to taste

1 whole lemon (sliced in quarters)
1 medium sized package of Spring salad mix

Sprinkle fresh ground pepper in a plate and lay tuna steak on top and turn until it is fully covered with pepper. Grill tuna approximately 3-4 minutes at high temperature until exterior of tuna steak is seared and cooked to your preference.

Cut seared tuna into 1" x 1" pieces and serve over the fresh spring salad. Top with sliced avocado and dried cranberries to taste. Season with soy sauce and lemon.

Basil-Almond Encrusted Flounder. For those who enjoy fish, this is a great dish that combines a white fish with basil and almonds for a delightful taste treat. Best of all it's a simple dish to make.

Simply grind a quarter cup of almonds in a food processor and chop up a half a cup of fresh basil. Now lay your fish on a piece of waxed paper and pour the almonds and basil over it. Rub them all over the flounder, turning it over in the mixture until it is fully covered. Saute in a frying pan using olive oil until each piece of fish is fully cooked. Serve with string beans and whole grained rice for an excellent dish. Another way to cook this dish is to broil it so that you do away with the oil altogether.

Trout Almondine. Follow the above instructions exchanging trout for flounder and only using the almonds. If you want to add a nice little change of pace to the taste, you may add a little almond and vanilla extracts to the olive oil as you are placing it in the pan. Or you can broil this dish to use less oil while cooking.

Shrimp. Shrimp are one of the easiest of all foods to prepare and they are tasty and filled with protein. You can simply cook them in boiling hot water until they are opaque, which is usually for about 3-5 minutes depending upon how large they are. Of course, the larger the shrimp, the longer it takes for them to be fully cooked. It is best to not eat uncooked or undercooked shrimp.

Shrimp Scampi. This is a richly flavored dish that normally features lots of butter and garlic and sauteed shrimp. It is not usually thought of as a "low calorie" dish. However, it is included because it is so tasty and you are able to substitute olive oil for the butter and use a butter substitute for flavoring purposes. You may also want to add some shallots and white wine to add a certain touch of elegance to the flavor of the dish. Of course, fresh squeezed lemon juice and fresh herbs will also add some zest to the dish. This dish can be the main course or it can act as a large appetizer depending upon your main course. Serves 8.

Ingredients:
24 large shrimp, shelled and de-veined, about 1 1/2 pounds
1/4 teaspoon sea salt
3 tablespoon extra virgin olive oil
3 1/2 tablespoon minced garlic
1 tablespoon unsalted butter or butter substitute
1/3 cup minced shallots (optional)
2 cups dry white wine (optional)
2 full lemons, juiced
2 teaspoon snipped fresh thyme
1 tablespoon finely chopped flat-leaf parsley

Sprinkle freshly washed shrimp with 1/2 teaspoon sea salt and set aside. Heat a large frying pan at medium heat and add the butter and olive oil. Add garlic and cook and stir for 1 minute. Add shallots and cook and stir until tender, about 3 minutes. Add seasoned shrimp, wine, lemon juice, and 1/2 teaspoon salt; bring to boiling.

Reduce heat and simmer, uncovered, for 2 to 3 minutes or until shrimp turn opaque, stirring occasionally. Remove shrimp with a slotted spoon; cover and keep warm.

Continue to gently boil liquid in skillet, uncovered, about 15 minutes or until liquid is slightly thickened and reduced to about 1 cup. Stir in parsley and thyme. Return shrimp to skillet and toss gently to coat with liquid in skillet. Transfer to a serving dish; serve warm.

Shrimp Kebabs. This is a wonderful way to use shrimp and vegetables together in an easy preparation. Serves 4.

Ingredients:
1/2 pound of shrimp pre-cooked and de-veined
2 Green peppers, sliced and cut in eighths
2 potatoes, peeled and cut into eighths
2 onions quartered
12 cherry tomatoes or two small tomatoes quartered

Using metal skewers, push the shrimp and all other ingredients onto each skewer, alternating each ingredient. Place on a barbeque or grill until fully cooked and serve. You may wish to add a little paprika and or garlic salt for taste. A fast and easy meal.

VEGETARIAN DISHES

If you truly want to lose weight or keep any additional pounds off your body, going primarily vegetarian is the best way to go. In fact, if you want to rehabilitate your arteries, vegetarian is the best way to go. So here are a few vegetarian dishes to get you started.

Steamed Vegetables and Thai Peanut Sauce. This is an easy to make and low calorie dish that tastes great. You can make it as spicy as you like. Serves 3-4.

Ingredients:
4 large unpeeled potatoes, sliced into 1/4 inch slices
2-3 large carrots, sliced into 1/4 inch slices
8 ounce package of fermented tofu (baked), sliced into 1/2"x1" squares
1medium sized broccoli, sliced into 1" sections
4 ounces green beans diagonally sliced into 1 1/2" sections

Thai Peanut Sauce:
1/2 cup peanut butter
1 tablespoon soy sauce
1 teaspoon chili paste or powder (to taste)

In a steamer, layer the potatoes and allow them to steam for approximately 4 minutes. Next layer in the opposing direction the carrots and let them steam for approximately 7 minutes more. Remove the carrots and potatoes and place on a platter and cover with a lid.

Now place the broccoli, green beans and tofu into the steamer and let them steam for an additional 4 minutes or until the vegetables are tender. Add the rest of the vegetables to the platter in an attractive arrangement and serve with the peanut sauce. Reserve 1/2 cup of the water from the steamer to make the sauce.

In a medium sized bowl, combine the sauce ingredients with 1/2 cup of reserved steaming liquid and whisk until smooth. Season with salt and pepper to taste. Serve in small bowls next to each dinner plate for dipping.

Spring Vegetables with Whole Wheat Pasta. This is a great spring dish that takes advantage of all the great fresh vegetables in season. Serves 4.

Ingredients:
3 1/2 cups of fresh or frozen vegetables of your choice. It is suggested you use baby carrots, spring onions, peas, asparagus and squash all cut up to 1-2" sections so they will cook quickly.
2 tablespoon butter
1 small clove of garlic, crushed
salt and pepper to taste
1/2 box of whole wheat pasta

Prepare whole wheat pasta according to the package directions and set aside. Steam the vegetables until done to your taste and toss with the pasta, melted butter and garlic. Season with salt and pepper to taste. You can also saute the vegetables and garlic in the butter until done and toss with pasta and season with salt and pepper to taste.

Black Bean Veggie-Burgers. Here's a great way to give yourself and your family "hamburgers" and still make them out of vegetables. This is a great quick and easy dish for summer cook-outs. The best part is it's all vegetables and low in calories but big on taste and texture. Serves 4.

Ingredients:
2 large cloves of chopped garlic
15 oz. can of black beans, rinsed and drained
1 large egg, whisked
2 large cloves of garlic
3 tablespoon olive oil
1/2 cup chopped cilantro
1/2 cup sliced scallions
1/2 cup finely chopped small chile pepper
1/2 cup of bread crumbs (whole wheat preferred)
1/2 teaspoon chili powder
1/2 teaspoon ground cumin
1/2 teaspoon salt

Heat a 10" skillet with a tablespoon of oil using medium heat and add the pepper, scallions and garlic until soft and cooked. Transfer vegetables to a food processor and pulse it 2-3 times until it is coarsely mixed but not too finely chopped. Pour into a bowl and mix in the rest of the contents (except for the remaining olive oil which will be used for cooking) and using your hands, make them into 4 veggie-burgers and then place them on a cooking sheet and refrigerate for at least a half hour and up to 5 hours. Cook like normal hamburgers in a pan (not on a grill please - they may fall apart), only using a little less heat and a little less time and serve. You may add a fruit salsa such as peach salsa and/or a guacamole dressing to add spice and interest to the dish. You may want to use whole wheat hamburger roles to the dish for consistency.

"Smoky" Corn Salsa. This is a great recipe because it makes enough to serve for a few days. It is great over chicken, fish or meat and can also be used in wraps and for dipping chips.

Ingredients:
2 red bell peppers, quartered & seeded
3-4 ears of fresh corn
1 bunch green onions
4 tablespoon olive oil
2 garlic cloves, diced
1 tablespoon bottled hot sauce
2 tablespoon fresh lime juice
1 teaspoon ground cumin
1/2 cup chopped fresh cilantro

Grill the peppers, onions and corm on an open grill at high heat for a short time or until they are a little charred. Make sure to cover them with olive oil before grilling so they will not stick to the grill. That will usually take between 5-15 minutes depending upon heat level. Slice the peppers and onions into 1/4 - 1/2 " squares. Cut the corn off the cob and set aside.

Now heat the firsts 2 tablespoons of olive oil in a frying pan over medium heat. Add garlic and cumin and cook for about 25-40 seconds. Pour contents into a large bowl and add lime juice and hot sauce to taste. Add the cooked vegetables. Add seasoning to taste and cool completely and then add the cilantro and mix in. Serve over meat, fowl, in wraps and as a dip for chips.

Vegetable Kebabs. This is a wonderful way to use shrimp and vegetables together in an easy preparation. Serves 4.

Ingredients:
1 broccoli, cut into 2" sections
2 green peppers, sliced and cut in eighths
2 potatoes, peeled and cut into eighths

2 onions quartered

12 cherry tomatoes or two small tomatoes quartered

Using metal skewers, push the broccoli and all other ingredients onto each skewer, alternating each ingredient. Place on a grill until desired doneness and serve. You may wish to add a little paprika, lemon juice and or garlic salt for taste. A fast and easy meal that is nutritious and low in calories.

Southern Oat Stuffed Peppers. Not only are these delicious, they also have a great deal of healing benefits. Oats have been found to assist your immune system, especially during cold and flu seasons.

Ingredients:
2 cups vegetable broth

2 cups cooked turkey sausage

1 chopped green pepper

1/4 cup oats

2 green peppers, cut in half

shredded mozzarella, to taste

Place vegetable broth in a soup pot and simmer, adding the cooked turkey sausage and chopped green pepper and bring to a boil. Add in oats and simmer for 5 minutes until it becomes thick. Allow mixture to cool. Stuff the green pepper halves with the cooled stuffing mixture and sprinkle mozzarella on top. Place in a heated oven at 350 degrees for 5 minutes. Serve hot with a bit of green garnish on top of each one.

SOMETIMES SIDE DISHES MATTER MOST

Here are a number of vegetable "side dishes" that you will often find in restaurants and diners as an adjunct to main courses. They are included to give you an idea of what they are and how to prepare them so you can fill out your main courses and yet not add a lot of calories or complex carbohydrates to your meal.

Asparagus. While seasonal in nature, asparagus is a good addition to almost any dish. While it has not been clinically substantiated, it appears that asparagus may have certain healing characteristics and is definitely an anti-oxidant. It offsets oxidizing factors in the blood. This can be very beneficial for you and your body as you return it to health after all your time smoking. It also makes your urine smell distinctively different, which not so subtly confirms you have recently eaten it. Best of all, there are many recipes available that use asparagus in them and they are all very tasty.

Baked Beans. These are normally purchased prepared and packaged in glass jars or cans (I prefer the jars). They are especially easy to prepare and go well with any barbeque and are a great side dish for so many entrees that it can be a staple of living. Beans are nutritious and healthful and taste great when served hot and are still good served cold.

Beets. Beets are a root, similar to carrots, and they cook up easily and add a wonderful red color to any dish. They are nutritious and healthful to eat. They can be either sweet or a little bitter, depending upon how you prepare them. They can be shredded or sliced and served with deviled eggs in a cold salad.

Broccoli. One of the very best foods you can eat. It has the highest energy content and contains lots of roughage to keep you feeling fuller longer. As a result of the fiber taking longer to digest, it will help you maintain your blood sugar at the right levels and help your digestive system move better throughout the day.

Broccoli Rabe. It is extremely high in nutrients and with the addition of raw crushed garlic in a sauce pan with a little olive oil, it will taste exquisite and give you plenty of nutrients and roughage as well, which, again, allows your blood sugar to stay high longer.

Brussels Sprouts. These are like small cabbages that are boiled or steamed and they contain great amounts of nutritious vitamins and fresh green roughage for your diet. Add a little garlic and they taste even better.

Cabbage. Cabbage can be used in a number of ways. It can be sliced and diced to be used in salads or cole slaw and it can be cooked after being quartered and added to corned beef for a favorite Irish dish of corned beef and cabbage. It can also be used as a simple addition to any other main dish and will add roughage and nutrients to your mean and give your body plenty to do for hours to come as it digests it and keeps you feeling full for a longer period of time.

Celery. A great base for dips, salsa and other toppings. You can use celery as an appetizer, snack or side dish. It is low in calories but high in fiber which means you won't feel hungry for awhile after eating it.

Cauliflower. This vegetable looks a lot like white broccoli in shape and is somewhat similar, but has different uses and nutrients. One of the best dishes to use cauliflower for is mashed cauliflower, a substitute for mashed potatoes. By whipping them up as if they were potatoes and adding some butter substitute and salt, they become better than mashed potatoes because they look and feel very much the same, but don't contain the complex carbohydrates that potatoes have in them.

Carrots. Fresh carrots are a great addition to any meal. Fresh carrots are filled with nutrients such as beta carotene and will add wonderful color to any dish. They are a root, so they offer additional nutrients that many other vegetables don't. You may either buy them prepared and sliced and fresh frozen or you may choose to buy them fresh and slice them yourself. If you buy fresh carrots, remember, the greens on top can sometimes be used as garnish on various dishes if it is relatively fresh and holds its shape. You can slice carrots along their length and use them as appetizers with a dip or you can simply chop them up along their length and boil or steam them until they are relatively soft and easy to eat.

Green Beans. These can be a great addition to any meal because they not only provide additional green vegetables to your meal, but they are tasty and nutritious as well. You can buy these fresh frozen and fully prepared in your grocery and all you need do is follow the directions on the side of the package. If you want to use fresh green beans, then cut off the stems and the very tip of the beans, drop them into boiling water and let them boil for no more than 5-7 minutes. Otherwise, they may overcook and lose their color, shape and nutritional value. Serve immediately after cooking.

Green Peas. Green peas are perhaps the easiest dish to make. Simply buy quick frozen green peas (I prefer the baby peas because they're sweeter), drop them into boiling water for just a few minutes and serve. Remember, if you're serving pasta or another dish that needs to be boiled, drop your peas into the dish just a minute or two before taking everything out of the boiling water and the peas will stay firm and nutritious rather than becoming boiled out from being in the water too long. If peas stay in boiling water more than 1-3 minutes, they tend to lose their color, firmness and nutritional value.

Kale. You can cook kale just like spinach. Either boil or steam it until it is fully softened and serve with as much fresh, crushed garlic as you like to taste. It is extremely good for you and with plenty of garlic, it tastes good too - especially if you like garlic.

Onions. These are a great low calorie addition to any dish and are easy to prepare fresh or you can find them in your frozen food department of your grocery store. If you're going to buy frozen, make sure there are no heavy sauces on the vegetables because that is usually where all the hidden calories are located. You may find "pearl onions" in prepared green pea packages and they add a nice change of flavor, however, it's probably best to stay away from "creamed onions" since they have a heavier cream base that is filled with calories and fat content. They are also great when they're fresh and used as part of a salad, chopped or sliced. They also come sliced or diced for a welcome addition to hamburgers, chicken and almost any kind of wrap, soup or salad.

Red Cabbage. A great dish to add to just about any meal. It is high in roughage and adds some color to what otherwise might be a bland looking dish. You can buy this prepared in a jar and simply heat it or you can simply buy it raw, slice it up in 1/4" strips and cook it to taste.

Spinach. While this may not initially be your favorite as a child, it can be made a lot better than when its simply boiled and served hot. Consider steaming raw spinach until it is wilted and then add garlic and other spices to taste and see how much more you enjoy it.

Squash. There are a number of types of squash available and it will depend upon the type you choose that will determine how you cook it. I like simplicity, so the easiest to make is Acorn Squash, which actually looks like a big green acorn.

To make Acorn Squash you first cut the squash in half midway from top to bottom after first cutting off the stem. The top of the squash is where the stem emerges from the squash. Next, scoop all seeds and loose "debris" from inside the squash, leaving the meaty sides intact. Place the two halves on a baking dish or pan, brush on some butter or butter substitute and sprinkle some cinnamon and brown sugar over it. You may wish to substitute Stevia FOS for the brown sugar which will work too. Place on a non-metallic plate or sheet and insert into a microwave and set it on high and run for approximately 15 minutes.

Depending upon differences in size, you may want to interrupt the microwave cycle a couple of times just to make sure the squash is fully cooked. Check it with a fork to see if it easily pokes through the meat of the squash. If not, put it in for another two minute interval and repeat the process until it is fully cooked and soft to the touch.

The preferred technique is to bake them without using a microwave by using a metallic sheet under the squash (and/or using aluminum foil to protect from spillage) and put it into a 350 degree oven and bake for approximately 30 minutes. Again, always check repeatedly to see if its fully cooked, since the timing will depend upon the variations in size of each squash.

Other types of squash can be done in a similar fashion, however, in those instances where squash is long and more narrow, the best approach is to split it down the middle, top to bottom and scoop out the innards and use similar spices and butter and do about the same procedure.

Tomatoes. Tomatoes are the basis of so many dishes, it's hard to imagine eating without this great vegetable. Tomatoes are an integral part of most salad, either quartered or whole if they are cherry tomatoes. One of the best dishes as a side dish is stewed tomatoes or you can simply place tomatoes in vinegar and sweetener and allow them to marinate for awhile and serve them as a cold dish for summery evening meals.

DESSERTS

While it's important to keep your weight stable after you quit smoking or even lose a little weight, it is just as important to not deny yourself those things you really enjoy in life. If you are one of the many people who enjoy desserts, here are a few suggestions that will help you maintain your weight or even lose some weight, yet still enjoy the sweetness you often crave at the end of a meal.

We've included not only low calorie desserts that you can have any time, but also a few desserts to really splurge as long as you cut back elsewhere on your caloric intake beforehand and afterward. What's the point of living if you can't enjoy yourself, right?

Fresh Fruit. This is one of the very best alternatives of all because you can use the freshest ingredients which contain the most and best nutrients for you. They're also basically low calorie and even when they have sugar in them, it's natural and the best type for your metabolism. The best part is when you eat fruit that is "in season," you also usually pay less for it and there is more of it available. One great place to but fresh and frozen produce is at Costco and other wholesale clubs. They appear to have the freshest produce and the lowest prices. Of course, you have to buy in bulk amounts but if you're following the advice in this book, you'll be eating more fruits and vegetables daily anyway and having a lot of them on hand will give you an incentive to eat them.

Here are some great additional recipes. You can augment them with spices, coverings and garnishes to make them more tasty and more eye appealing as you wish.

Low-Cal Sherbert. Most supermarkets now have low calorie sherberts available, however, even if it isn't lo-cal, it's far better for you and your body than ice cream or other desserts. Even those sherbets with sugar as their first ingredient are still better than ice cream.

Another way to enjoy any type of sherbert you want is to make it yourself. The best way to do that is to take any type of frozen berries, strawberries, raspberries, blueberries, blackberries, etc. and place them into your blender with a little water. How much water is up to your tastes. This is somewhat experimental, so be prepared to vary the amounts to your needs. Add Stevia with FOS (see appendix for natural sweeteners for an explanation) to augment the natural sweetness of the berries. Blend to the consistency you like. Be aware that the consistency will usually be more watery than you might want it to be, but it will be fine once it is frozen. Take the mixture and freeze to the consistency you like, slushy, watery, ice cube and anything in between. Serve in individual dessert bowls with a little mint leaf for garnish and you'll enjoy a low calorie, natural dessert.

Low Calorie Jello. While this may seem a little mundane to many, it still makes a great dessert and is low in calories if you use the lo-cal type. Of course, even if you use the regular Jello, it's still not all that heavy on the calories so it makes a great treat at the end of a meal without adding fat or complex carbohydrates.

Balsamic Sabayon Over Berries. This is a great dish to have with any kind of berries, strawberries, raspberries, blueberries, blackberries, etc. It tastes wonderful and still doesn't have to be too high in calories or sugar. To have less calories, use Stevia with FOS (see appendix for natural sweeteners for an explanation), honey or maple syrup for sweetness and fewer calories.

It is important to make the sabayon the day you intend upon serving it, although it may last an extra day if absolutely necessary. Start by whisking 4 egg yolks and the equivalent of 6 tablespoons of unrefined or brown sugar or the equivalent of Stevia FOS in a small stainless steel bowl until it is completely combined. You will know by when the coloring turns lighter. Then immerse the bowl in a pan of simmering hot water while you continue to whisk the mixture until it thickens.

You'll know the mixture is cooked when it turns light and it leaves long strings as you lift your whisk out of the mixture. Beware of overcooking or you can ruin the outcome. After removing it from the heat, place the bowl over a larger bowl filled with ice and now whisk in 2 tablespoons of clear balsamic vinegar. Continue for about 5-8 minutes until the mixture is fully cooled. Whip 1 1/2 cups of whipping cream until it is slightly thickened and then gently fold it into the cooled mixture. Once fully mixed, refrigerate for at least 2 hours before serving.

Now prepare your berries by first washing them thoroughly, coring them and slicing them thinly. Serve them in clear glass dessert dishes with a garnish of mint leaves picked from your garden and you have an exquisite dessert. Of course, this is another one of those that can only be eaten a few times a year, but it will be well worth the wait.

Strawberry Shortcake. This is one of many people's favorites, but also one of the worst for keeping weight off, so don't eat it more than 3 or 4 times a year. That will also keep it special and something to look forward to at special times. As a kid I liked it so much that I declared that I was in charge of making it for everyone and I still do so to this day.

It is very simple and easy to make and if you don't use too much whipped cream, it's not that high in calories, carbohydrates or fat. Remember this should be one of those few desserts you treat yourself with only from time to time when you've eliminated all desserts from your menu for a week or two.

Ingredients:
1 sleeve of biscuits from the refrigerated section
1 pint of frozen strawberries in heavy syrup
1 1/2 pint of heavy whipping cream
1/2 tsp of vanilla extract
1/4 tsp of almond extract
Add Stevia to taste

Thaw the strawberries and prepare biscuits according to the package directions. Whip the cream, adding the sweeter and extracts slowly. Whip until soft peaks form when you lift the beater up.

If you want to eliminate the heavy sugary syrup (and you should), pour off all the syrup from the strawberries, rinse and drain. Take a portion of the strawberries and puree in a blender and add Stevia until you get the right amount of sweetness for you. Mix with the remaining strawberries. If you don't really have a sweet tooth, you can use fresh sliced strawberries and the whipped cream as a filler instead.

Split a biscuit with a fork and place 1 half on a plate and spoon the strawberries on top (or layer if you are using fresh sliced strawberries). Cover with the other biscuit half and drop a dollop of whipped cream onto the top. Top with a strawberry and drizzle a little strawberry syrup over the top so it runs down the sides. You'll love it and look forward to it once every 3-4 months or at holiday time.

Apricot Yogurt. This is a great way to eat a relatively low calorie flavored yogurt that not only tastes good, but is good for you. It reinstates the good flora into your intestines. Serves 2.

Ingredients:
1 1/2 cups plain live culture low fat yogurt
1/4 cup apricot syrup
1 dried apricot half
1/4 cup evaporated skim milk

Combine the yogurt, evaporated milk and apricot syrup in a medium sized bowl and stir until the mixture is smooth. Spoon into individual dessert dishes. Then slice and dice the apricot half and sprinkle it over the mix and serve chilled with a mint leaf for garnish.

Mandarin Orange Yogurt. This is basically the same dish as the apricot yogurt, except you change the fruit ingredient. You add 2 teaspoons of orange marmalade, 1/2 teaspoon of orange extract and 1/4 cup of drained mandarin oranges to the mix. Follow the same directions as for Apricot Yogurt and exchange the Mandarin Oranges, marmalade and extract for the Apricots. Or, you can simply add the two together for an additional taste treat.

Mango Yogurt. Use the same basic recipe from the Apricot Yogurt and substitute fresh Mango for the Apricot and you have yet another tasty treat.

Fruit Yogurt Over Fresh Fruit. Now that you know how to make various fruit yogurt, it's time to combine them with fresh berries when they are in season and other fresh fruits such as cherries, peaches, pears, plums and anything else that catches your eye and your imagination. Simply divide up the fresh fruit you have into individual dessert cups or bowls and pour your fruit yogurt over it to add to the overall taste and texture. It's a great dessert to serve after a meal.

Peach Popover. This is a great dessert and it is low in calories.

Ingredients:
1/3 cup regular flour
3 tablespoons whole wheat flour
1/2 cup skim milk
1 egg
1 tablespoon brown sugar
1/4 teaspoon cinnamon
1/8 teaspoon salt
1 tablespoon butter or butter substitute like olive oil
1 large sized fresh peach, washed, peeled and sliced

Mix the brown sugar and cinnamon and set aside in a small bowl. Beat the egg in a medium sized bowl until it is fluffy and then add in the regular and whole wheat flour, together with the milk and salt. Preheat a 9" or 10" ceramic or metal pie pan at 400 degrees and once heated, take out and cover the bottom with the butter or oil. Make sure the entire pan is covered, including the sides. Now pour the batter into the pre-heated pie pan and arrange the sliced peaches around the entire pie pan. Sprinkle the brown sugar/cinnamon mixture over the entire mixture. Return the pan to the oven and allow to cook until it rises up and is brown and puffy, approximately 25 minutes. Remove and serve hot by slicing it like a pizza. It goes especially well with a meat or poultry dish for a main meal.

Cherry Cluster Pudding. Here's a great way to use naturally sweet pitted cherries into a pudding that will make your mouth water while preparing it. Serves 4.

Ingredients:
1 cup frozen unsweetened cherries (pitted)
1 cup skim milk
1 envelope of unflavored gelatin (1/4 oz.)
1/4 cup of cold water
1 teaspoon almond extract
1/2 teaspoon Vanilla extract

Defrost the cherries and choose 2 for the "Cherry on Top" and set aside for later. Cut the remaining cherries in half and return them to the freezer until needed.

Stir the gelatin and cold water in a small bowl and let sit for 3 minutes to soften. Heat the skim milk in a saucepan until it bubbles around the edge. Pour the heated milk into the gelatin and stir until the gelatin is completely dissolved, cover tightly. Place in the refrigerator for 20-30 minutes until it has starts to get thicker. Whip with a whisk or beater until fluffy.

Puree the thawed cherries (except for the toppings) and pour through a strainer to eliminate any pieces of skin or cherry meat that is still not pureed. Now add the cherry puree to the gelatin mixture and add the almond and vanilla extracts and stir until thoroughly mixed. Pour into four dessert bowls and add the cherry halves that you've saved in the freezer and refrigerate for a minimum of 4 hours and up to overnight. Serve fully chilled. Each serving is less than 65 calories.

HEALTHY LOW CALORIE SNACKS

Here are some great snacks to keep you fat free and give you a boost at the same time. Notice there are no sweets or crackers in the mix. All the suggestions are wholesome and nutritious and taste great at the same time. This is an excellent opportunity to retrain your mind to love good food that is good for you as well.

Applesauce Celery Sticks. These are a healthier alternative to celery sticks with peanut butter that are very low in calories yet they give you a little natural sweetness to go with the celery flavor. Use natural unsweetened applesauce if you want to further reduce your sugar intake.

Avocado/Turkey Wrap. This is another low fat, high protein snack that will taste great and give you energy. Wrap three slices of Avocado in a slice of fresh turkey with a little dab of mustard. Instead of using the bread, use a large leaf of Romaine lettuce. Low calorie and high in green content which contains great nutrients to de-acidify your internal body chemistry.

Breadless Low Fat BLT Wrap. Wrap a slice of sliced fresh turkey, two slices of avocado, a slice of low fat cheese and a generous dab of mustard in a large leaf of Romaine lettuce and serve.

Cheese Filled Tomatoes. These look as good as they taste and they're simple to make. Simply cut the tops off of 4 small/medium tomatoes and scoop out the innards. Fill with a mixture of 1/2 cup of cottage cheese or ricotta cheese mixed with 1/2 cup of plain unsweetened yogurt.

Tuna Salad Filled Tomatoes. Same as the cheese filled tomatoes, but filled with tuna salad made with brown or yellow mustard to keep the calories and fat content low.

Chicken Salad Filled Tomatoes. Of course, the same as the cheese filled and tuna tomatoes, but using leftover chicken that you didn't eat when you cooked your full chicken at a previous meal.

Peanut Butter Celery Sticks. This is a real snack time treat since it has peanut butter in it along with celery, which is both filling and provides a small amount of "green" to your diet. Plus, it has plenty of roughage in it to add to the time it takes to be fully digested by your body, keeping your blood sugar more stable. The one down side of this treat is that peanut butter is mostly fat from nuts and usually has some sugar in it. The best type of peanut butter to use is natural peanut butter that has no hydrogenated or poly-unsaturated oils in it. There are now peanut butter brands that use maple sugar in them as a substitute for sugar and that's the one I use and recommend.

Sauteed Shrimp. Use the rest of your shrimp and saute them in trans-fat free olive oil. Add hot sauce and some oregano and/or paprika and serve them hot or cold.

Shrimp Cocktail. While this may sound like an expensive "snack," it's not all that expensive and is very low in calories and fat. Simply buy a pound or two of frozen shrimp and use 1/4 pound for a serving for two. Defrost, de-vein and cook what you want to eat and serve on a plate with a small custard cup of pre-made cocktail sauce, a few slices of lemon and a basil leaf or the greens from fresh carrots on the side. You'll feel like you're living it up and not gaining any weight at the same time.

Tuna Celery Sticks. This is a great way to have a low fat snack and eat some great fiber at the same time. Mix a can of tuna fish with a tablespoon of brown mustard to taste. Add some additional lemon juice and a splash of low fat/low sugar Italian dressing and mix. Fill 4" long celery sticks with the mixture and serve. The same thing can be done with chicken for a slightly different taste.

Turkey Roll-Ups. Fill a slice of fresh cut smoked turkey with sweet pepper sticks, a slice of low fat Jarlsberg cheese and a hearty dab of mustard.

LAST THOUGHTS ON FOODS AND RECIPES

Anyone can give you advice on how to make low calorie food or low fat food, but the decisive factor of whether or not you maintain or lose weight is simply how much you eat and what you eat. If you are mindful of everything you eat - as you eat it - you will likely never gain any weight after quitting smoking. If you sit in front of the television and eat mindlessly or eat whenever you're stressed, unhappy, tired or angry, you'll be far more likely to gain weight over time.

The real essence of maintaining your weight is to plan what you're going to eat, using nutritious, healthy choices and eat a number of meals daily, rather than just two or three meals. Make sure you end all eating by 7 PM and you'll begin to notice that you start losing weight quickly and easily almost effortlessly. Follow the recipes and suggestions in this book, especially those that help you use Emotional Freedom Technique to obliterate your food craving and you'll notice major changes in your eating habits.

The long and short of the entire issue comes down to you and how seriously you want to maintain your weight or lose weight. Of course, exercise always plays an important part in the overall strategy of losing weight and its best to simply keep to a steady regimen of aerobic exercise to keep your metabolism pumping and automatically burning off calories.

In the long run, the best part of the entire equation is you've become a non-smoker for life and that will add years to your life. Now if you maintain or even lose weight, you'll feel much better at the same time.

Congratulations!! You're a non-smoker for life!

CHAPTER 6

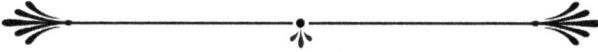

SOME FOOD AND EXERCISE CLARIFICATIONS

FOOD MISUNDERSTANDINGS

There are often many misunderstandings about food and its effect upon your body and your health. Many of these are so well known that many still hang on to them tenaciously even when they've been proven untrue. Here are some of those typical misunderstandings about food for you to consider.

Carbohydrates are bad for you - Not True!

Many diets in the past (like the Atkins Diet) have claimed that if you cut out all carbohydrates, you'll lose weight. While that's often true, it's not the entire story. Carbohydrates play an important and strategic role in keeping your energy up and keeping your organs functioning properly. You need carbohydrates in order to get enough energy into your body to keep everything running smoothly. Otherwise, you'll likely feel empty and lacking in energy.

When nutritionists say to stay away from carbohydrates and define them as "everything white" they usually mean items such as white rice, white bread, white sugar, white pasta and sometimes white potatoes. That's because those carbohydrates tend to cause weight gain and fat accumulation within your body.

Instead of eating "white carbohydrates" you can easily substitute brown rice, whole wheat bread, 12 grain bread, whole wheat pasta and natural brown sugar. Just by doing this, you'll be changing the level of your "bad" carbohydrates dramatically and before long you'll notice you start to lose weight and start feeling better.

Margarine has less fat than butter - False!
A teaspoon of butter and a teaspoon of solid stick margarine have exactly the same amounts of fat (4 grams) and the same number of calories (36). However, butter has saturated fat, which is the primary cause of high cholesterol, while margarine contains trans fat, which is so unhealthy that it's been banned in most restaurants and even fast food places in the United States. Take your pick. My pick is butter over margarine every time. Not only does it taste better, in the long run it is much better for you as long as you only eat it in moderation. If you know it has a negative aspect to it, you can reduce the amount you eat and still get to enjoy it's taste and consistency.

If you want to know which is product is better for you to bake or cook with and you want to reduce the saturated fats in your diet, you might consider switching to soft tub or liquid margarine; many of which are now trans fat-free and reasonably low in saturated fat. For toast, use soft spreads or, even better, dip your bread into a little extra-virgin olive oil, which is one of the healthiest fats nature ever created.

If you want to use a oil for cooking, use Pam or other similar spray-on oils. You can also use olive oil which is one of the only oils that don't break down as much as all others under heat, plus it adds a nice taste and consistency to the dish you're cooking.

Overall, the medical profession and nutritionists generally recommend that healthy people should consume no more than approximately 200 milligrams of cholesterol daily. Bear in mind that butter has about 100 calories in each knife swipe of it and about 33 milligrams of cholesterol in one tablespoon, so if you're going to use butter, use it sparingly!

One suggestion to consider if you love your butter and don't want to let it go is to use whipped butter since it has more air in it. More air means less butter per spoonful. By using whipped butter you can reduce the normal number of grams of fat in regular bar butter from 11 grams down to 7 grams and you'll also reduce the saturated fat down from 8 grams down to roughly 5 grams.

While that still is high, its much better than the normal amount of fat grams and it will make a difference to your overall health than using regular hard butter.

Low-fat foods means low-calorie foods - Not Necessarily True!
While low fat is often a good indicator of less calories, the truth is that especially with processed foods, many food manufacturers actually increase fillers in order to reduce fat. Fillers are not very healthy - or low in calories. So, when you check the label, you may notice less fat content, but higher calories at the same time.

As an example, natural peanut butter contains a high amount of peanut oil which contains fat - which means more fat intake. However, regular popular brands of peanut butter contain less natural fat, but in order to make their product creamy (which is not the case with natural peanut butter) the manufacturers add sugary corn syrup and trans fat products (remember, the "bad" stuff) to keep it creamy. Bad idea, but most people like their peanut butter creamy and really don't notice the labels. Another bad idea.

Instead of staying with the popular brands that have all that very bad trans fat and corn syrup within them, switch to natural peanut butter and stir it up yourself and just spread it thinner than usual. That way, you still keep the taste, but limit the amount of your peanut oil intake and you get the best of both worlds and you reduce your caloric intake.

Whole eggs increase your cholesterol count - Not True!
Actually, whole eggs are better for you than egg whites alone. This issue has often been misunderstood which is almost entirely wrong. Eggs are known for their low calories and high protein content. They are also high in vitamins B12, D, Folic Acid. This myth has been around for many, many years to the point that many diet conscious people only eat "egg white" omelettes because they believe egg

whites better for them. Actually, nothing could be more wrong. Egg yolks actually help dissipate the "bad" cholesterol in the body.

Remember, cholesterol is made by the body from within the body and we need various cholesterol limiting chemicals - via food - to curtail their negative effects. Whole eggs are a great source of such chemicals. In fact, medical research has recently verified that the mixture of various fats you eat are what primarily contribute to the "bad" cholesterol in your body rather than your intake of fat alone.

As a practical matter, have your cholesterol checked and see where it is on the normal scale before eating whole eggs on a regular basis. If you're in the normal range (HDL above 45 mg/dl, LDL below 100), then go ahead and enjoy your daily egg or even a couple of omelettes a week. Remember, eggs alone are not the real problem in your diet.

When all else fails, use the grapefruit diet - False!
Versions of this "diet" have been around for decades. They usually are all about eating very few calories of primarily high protein and adding grapefruit for as long as you can stand eating it. If you followed that regimen consistently for a long time, you will very likely lose weight, but you would more than likely put it all back on as soon as you stopped the "diet." Instead of "dieting," you may want to consider a simple life style change that remains a permanent fixture in your daily life such as ending your "addiction" to sweets and/or chips and dips.

On the other hand, grapefruit can play an important role in your dietary intake if you use it correctly. Instead of reducing your carbs and substituting grapefruit, why not simply add a half a grapefruit or a glass of grapefruit juice at each meal? This will do two things for you. First, it will add natural Vitamin C to your diet and that will help alkalize your body chemistry. That can be a very good thing, especially for former smokers because their bodies have been "acidified" as a result of smoking for many years and an acidic internal environment is the breeding ground for cancer. So by alkalizing your body chemistry, you lessen the likelihood of allowing cancer to grow within your body.

Second, grapefruit tends to "burn off" fat quicker than most foods because it contains certain plant chemicals and compounds that appear to lower insulin levels, which in turn, causes you to lose weight more easily. In fact, those who use this modified system of a half a grapefruit before each meal have lost about 1/2 a pound a week while they're doing it. After you've lost the amount of weight you want, then you may consider modifying your grapefruit intake to alternating meals or days until you normalize your intake again.

EXERCISING MISUNDERSTANDINGS

If you don't sweat, your workout is worthless - Simply Not True! Most people who workout believe that for it to be useful, you have to sweat and get winded. While those types of workouts can be very beneficial and help you keep your body healthy, a less impact causing workout can be just as beneficial. A low-impact workout, like brisk walking, yoga, stretching and light weight-lifting are another important way to keeping your muscles active and strong and keep your metabolism burning calories all day long. This is especially so for those who are older and are worried that they haven't worked out for quite some time and they don't want to jump into it all at once.

First, make sure to have a medical checkup before starting any exercise regimen and get yourself cleared for working out.

Then, after you've done a moderate amount of low-impact workouts, then you can begin to include more rigorous cardiovascular workouts and weight or resistance training into your exercise regimen and you'll really start to see the full benefit of an overall workout.

Weight-Lifting Automatically Gives you Big Muscles - False!
While weight lifting can give men big muscles, women are less likely to build defined muscles that make them lose their feminine body shape because of three important factors. One, women have an extra layer of body fat that men don't have, which causes their muscles to look more rounded and not as "cut" as men's musculature. Two, women don't have as much testosterone in them as men do and so they have less propensity to build sharp edged muscles. Three, when either gender is working out with weights, if you want to tone up your muscles and not bulk them up, simply reduce the amount of weight you're lifting and increase the repetitions of lifting and your muscles will smooth out and become toned, without becoming huge and cut.

You may have Heard that Muscle Weighs More than Fat - False!
A pound of muscle and a pound of fat weigh the same - a pound is a pound either way! That's obvious. The real difference in them is the density of muscle is much more than fat and that's what most people are referring to when they say "I've been dieting and can't understand why I weight more now than before I started working out."

The truth is that many times people will initially gain some weight when they start working out because muscle is denser than fat and a lot less "jiggly" than fat. What most people who diet want is to eliminate the "jiggles" in various areas of their body and that can only be done by working out and toning the body's muscles, while at the same time eliminating their complex carbohydrate intake so that the body will start using up the fat that stores excess energy taken into the body in the past.

Hence, they start to tone up their muscles initially and it takes a little more time to eliminate the body fat that has been with them for awhile, so they initially put on weight and often use that as a rationale for quitting their exercise regimen instead of sticking with it until they see real results. In fact, muscle and fat weight the same, they just look very different on your body.

CONCLUSION

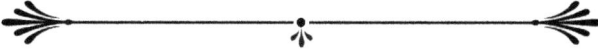

Don't forget one cardiologist's food plan advice: "If it tastes too good or too sweet - spit it out."

***

Some Additional Hopeful News about Quitting Smoking - Even If You Already Have Cancer

An article in the British Medical Journal, now known as BMJ, claimed that, for the first time, people who already have lung cancer, if they immediately quit, can as much as **double** their chances of survival. That's amazing!

Normally, people with lung cancer who kept smoking reportedly have about a 30% chance of surviving beyond five years. However, those who immediately quit smoking increased their chance of survival to 65% after five years.

Remember, lung cancer is the most prevalent form of cancer worldwide, and the potential for recovery is usually poor to very poor. Normally, if left undiagnosed and untreated, only about 7% of patients survive five years. Although about 20% of lung cancer patients are diagnosed early enough to be successfully treated and they survive longer.

The important message to remember is if you're a smoker, first get checked for lung cancer as often as possible and if you are diagnosed with lung cancer, quit smoking immediately. Actually, come to think of it, its even better if you simply quit now. However, "never give up on giving up (smoking)," said Amanda Parsons, of the U.K. Center for Tobacco Control Studies at the University of Birmingham, who led the study.

Ironically enough, it appears that not all medical doctors recommend immediately stopping smoking, even when their patients are diagnosed with lung cancer. They often claim that it only makes their patients feel worse and adds to their feelings of guilt because their smoking habit resulted in cancer which affects not only them, but their families as well. However, this was included in this book because it must change and doctors must learn to tell their patients and their families about the results of this study, because the potential benefit of quitting is too great to ignore.

The research also confirmed that it was not just the smoke or the nicotine that caused cancer, but both of them together speed the spread of lung cancer. It still appears that lung and all other cancers are initiated by the acidic environment caused by smoking and the inability to eliminate acids from the body, such as lactic acid, which is produced by muscular movement. This is because the pores of the skin become clogged by tar and other ingredients in cigarettes and the liver is unable to filter out those poisons as efficiently as before the smoker became a smoker. There is little clinical proof of this theory yet, however, it remains to be proven in the future.

Most importantly, it's a clear message that even if you have cancer, if you quit smoking immediately upon learning of it you double your chances of survival. Those are better odds than certain death. But the question arises - why wait until you develop cancer? Why not quit today and lessen your potential for cancer in the first place. That way, your percentages for eliminating cancer and lots of other diseases increase dramatically and best of all, you will start feeling better almost immediately.

As you can see, quitting smoking is just the start to improving your life. Once you are successful at quitting smoking, you will often experience a burst of energy, joy and excitement as you start to feel better physically and emotionally. You will also start to develop more self-confidence and greater self-esteem, which, in turn, will open new opportunities for you to improve your life and body in many other ways. In effect, once you realize you can accomplish what may have. at one time, seemed impossible, everything changes and new horizons become available to you. This is your opportunity to change your life in many ways. You'll be surprised at just how successful you can be in your life now that you've stopped smoking.

I trust these tips and techniques will help you remain slim while you learn to enjoy the benefit's of being a non-smoker for the rest of your life. Remaining slim will make your life that much better than it would be if you gained weight after quitting smoking. By changing a few of your eating habits and incorporating certain leafy green vegetables you will start to naturally reverse the harm done to your body while you smoked.

With the passage of time your lungs and body will start to regenerate and with a renewed interest in exercise, you'll find your body will become healthy again. By using the EFT regimen you will find you can not only help eliminate your urges to smoke or other bad habits, it will help you eliminate any negative emotions as well. All of this can occur while you stay slim and remain a non-smoker for the rest of your life.

I trust you will see the benefit's of following these simple techniques and will realize they have already started to help you change your life. If trying to implement all of them at once seems overwhelming, then do one at a time until you accumulate them all. You'll know you've "arrived" when you start noticing a real difference in how, and what you eat and how often. Continue to use the tips and techniques and watch how much better your life will be in the future.

If you have any ideas you'd like to suggest, please feel free to contact us and let us know.

Blessings,
Theodore W. Robinson

APPENDIX

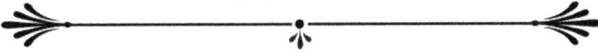

CALORIES IN ALCOHOLIC BEVERAGES

Some people want to give up smoking, but still enjoy drinking alcohol and don't want to give up their alcoholic drinks. While the admonition still applies that imbibing alcohol is fundamentally bad for your mind and will bloat your body, if you are intent upon drinking alcohol, then here are a few ideas on how to drink responsibly and enjoy it with less guilt. If you're going to imbibe, you might as well enjoy it as much as possible.

However, since the rest of this book is about becoming more conscious about what you do and what you put into your body, the following chart will provide you with the calories, fat and carbohydrates of a number of different drinks so you can make informed choices about what and how much you choose to imbibe.

The calories and carbohydrates aren't always consistent with one another, so you have to be mindful of what you drink. However, if you drink moderately, you should be able to keep your caloric intake in check. The definition of moderate drinking is no more than 2 drinks a day for men and 1 drink a day for women. A "drink" is considered a drink when you imbibe 12 ounces of beer, 5 ounces of wine or 1 1/2 ounces of 80 proof distilled liquor like scotch, vodka, gin, whiskey or rye. If you vary the amounts or mix the types of fluids, do your best to keep in mind how much you're drinking and how many calories and carbohydrates you're taking into your body and by keeping that in mind, you'll almost automatically drink in moderation.

Item	Serving Size	Carb. (grams)	Fat (grams)	Calories
Beer, light	12 oz.	6.9	0	110
Beer, regular	12 oz.	11.9	0	144
Cocktails: (carb. and fat depend on recipe used)				
Bacardi	2.5 oz.			120
Black Russian	3 oz.			245
Bloody Mary	5 oz.			116
Daiquiri	2 oz.			120
Gin & Tonic	7.5 oz.			165
Manhattan	2.5 oz.			130
Margarita	3 oz.			155
Martini	2.5 oz.			137
Mint Julep	10 oz.			215
Old Fashioned	4 oz.			180
Pina Colada	4.5 oz.			265
Screwdriver	7 oz.			175
Tom Collins	7.5 oz.			120
Whiskey Sour	3 oz.			125
White Russian	3.5 oz.			275
Distilled gin, rum, vodka, & whiskey (80 proof)	1 oz.	0	0	65
Liqueur, coffee (53 proof)	1 oz.	16	.1	118
Liqueur, creme de menthe (72 proof)	1 oz.	14	.1	127

Item	Serving Size	Carb. (grams)	Fat (grams)	Calories
Wine, red	1 wine glass (4 oz.)	1.7	0	91
Wine, white	1 wine glass (4 oz.)	1.7	0	86
Wine, rose	1 wine glass (4 oz.)	1.7	0	90
Wine, dessert	3 oz.	10.04	0	130
Wine, port	2 oz.	6	0	86

Note: Since I've also been a criminal defense lawyer for 36 years, I feel compelled to share this little tidbit with you. Whatever you do, if you intend upon drinking while you're out of your home, make sure you have a designated driver to drive your car. In this day and age, nobody is safe from a DWI, Driving While Intoxicated, or driving under the influence of alcohol DWAI if they've had as little as two drinks and even less than that if the police officer is interested in making an arrest. It's simply better to avoid the entire situation than trying to defend yourself especially when you're innocent. So do whatever is necessary to protect yourself from being arrested and at the same time, you're keeping your caloric intake down.

SWEETENERS - WHICH ARE BEST FOR YOU?

There has been so much written about refined sugar and how bad it is for your health. However, as time goes by it becomes increasingly obvious that most artificial sweeteners are even underline worse for you than sugar. We've supplied you with a list of the artificial sweeteners on the market right now and their overall "sweetness" rating to give you a better idea of what is available and then some commentary about which is best for you.

Suffice it to say all processed food, including refined sugar, is not as good for you as natural, organic or unprocessed food. Processing means that the food product has been changed from its original state by bleaching, crushing, powdering, homogenizing, pasteurizing, or even by being partially digested.

The artificial sweeteners are listed relative to the sweetness of sugar by weight to give you an idea of how little you would have to use in relation to how much sugar you would normally use. The trade names and manufacturer of each is included to give you some idea of how to locate it in stores. They also list whether they have been approved by the FDA or not to give you an idea of whether they're considered safe to eat. Notice that one has already been banned and is presently pending re-approval by the FDA.

Alitame
2,000 times the sweetness of sugar of sugar, Pending FDA Approval

Aspartame
160–200 times the sweetness of sugar, "NutraSweet", FDA Approved 1981

Cyclamate
30 times the sweetness of sugar, FDA Banned 1969, pending re-approval

Glucin
300 times the sweetness of sugar

Neohesperidin dihydrochalcone
1,500 times the sweetness of sugar

NutraSweet (Neotame)
8,000 times the sweetness of sugar, FDA Approved 2002

Nutrinova (Acesulfame potassium)
200 times the sweetness of sugar, FDA Approved 1988

Saccharin
300 times the sweetness of sugar, FDA Approved 1958

Splenda (Sucralose)
600 times the sweetness of sugar, FDA Approved 1998

Truvia
Marketed by CocaCola and PepsiCo, The FDA that it has no objection to their products, referring to them as "safe." Both come from an extract of the stevia plant which is good. Both have about zero calories in them.

Twinsweet (Salt of aspartame - acesulfame)
350 times the sweetness of sugar

While all diet sodas and many other drinks contain some sort of artificial sweetener which brings their calorie count as low as 1 or even down to zero, they are best avoided at all costs. From my own experience, they invariably appear to cause you to have more of an appetite rather than less and most leave a bad after-taste in your mouth and they generally not particularly good for you. This is my opinion only, however, from my own experience, I've noticed that when I have sugar-sweetened soft drinks, such as iced tea, I notice I have less negative after effects then when I drink artificially sweetened soft drinks. Your experience may be different, however, its simply best to stay with natural products as much as possible.

HEALTHY AND NATURAL SUGAR SUBSTITUTES

Remember, you don't need to live a life without the taste of sweetness. That's not the purpose of this book. There are plenty of natural choices available from which to choose. The following can be used to sweeten your coffee or tea as well as in baked goods.

Stevia which contains FOS

Stevia is a very sweet herb that's available in powder and/or liquid forms at health-food stores. FOS is an acronym for "fruit ogiliosaccharides," which support healthy intestinal bacteria, or flora, which are necessary for good health. When used together, Stevia with FOS is a non-nutritive powder that is not only exceptionally sweet, but also helpful to your digestive tract. However, be careful - only use a little at a time. Because it is so sweet, a little of it goes a long way.

Honey and Agave Nectar

Honey, especially single blossom honey like red clover honey or orange blossom honey, is a low-glycemic sweetener. It won't increase your blood sugar too dramatically when you eat it. You can comfortably use honey in all your beverages as well as baked goods. The same holds true for Agave nectar. However, both are high in calories and carbohydrates, so use them in moderation.

Xylitol

Xylitol, also called birch sugar, can be effectively used for baking and other sweetening purposes. It is also a low-glycemic sweetener. It generally won't cause blood sugar imbalances or yeast infections like table sugar often does. It will also help prevent tooth decay and plaque and will help improve your bone structure. One thing to note, however, is you should restrict your intake somewhat because if you overuse it, you may experience diarrhea and stomach cramps.

Fructose

Fructose is another natural low-glycemic impacting sugar that is derived from fruit. You will often find it in a granulated form in health-food stores. Fructose is somewhat sweeter than regular white sugar, so you will need less to get the same level of sweetness from it. However, if you ingest too much fructose by drinking syrupy sodas and beverages sweetened with high-fructose corn syrup, or eating processed foods such as syrups and candy that contain high-fructose corn syrup, it can increase the lipids in your body that then increase the potential for heart disease. So stay away from syrupy and sweet processed foods. However, it should be okay for you to eat all the fruit you want and use fructose sparingly as a sweetener.

Sucrose (White Refined Table Sugar)
White refined table sugar (sucrose), is a medium-glycemic sweetener and okay for most people if you only eat or drink small amounts, like sweetening your coffee or tea with a single portion (one cube or sugar packet). However, eating large amounts of refined sugar, such as in candy, soda and sweet baked goods, should be refrained from and not be a part of your food plan.

Brown Sugar
Another way to sweeten drinks and other things is to consider using brown unprocessed sugar instead of refined white sugar. It is much better for you and will have less negative effects upon you than almost any artificial sweetener or certainly less than refined or processed sugar of any kind.

Maple Syrup
Last, but not least, maple syrup is about as natural a sweetener as you can get. It comes directly from Sugar Maple trees in the North-eastern United States and Canada and is concentrated through various processes. It has a low glycemic index and is a great way to sweeten dishes without adding too many calories and generally, it is organically produced.

You can use all of these natural sweeteners with confidence, but always with restraint. Remember, everything is best used in moderation, especially sweeteners.

INDEX

NOTIFICATION AND WAIVER

The information contained in this booklet is presented for information purposes only. The material is in no way intended to replace professional medical or psychological care or attention by a qualified and licensed medical or mental health practitioner. While we believe that EFT works well with many symptoms, it is still theoretical and there is no universally accepted scientific explanation for its efficacy yet. The version of EFT we practice and teach is slightly different than that of Gary Craig, the developer of EFT.

Ted Robinson is an Interfaith spiritual minister. He practices and teaches EFT and is certified in hypnosis by the National Guild of Hypnotists. He is not a licenced therapist or health care professional in any area.

He believes that all healing has a spiritual basis and that ultimately everyone heals themselves. He does not offer any medical or psychological advice other than to advise all clients that they are always responsible for their own health care and if they feel they need medical or mental health care, they should consult with a medical or mental health care professional.

All readers are advised to obtain a waiver from their primary care or mental health care professional before utilizing EFT, Hypnosis or any other alternative health care. No client should discontinue or modify any prescriptive medication without obtaining prior medical approval. All clients assume all risk and responsibility for any adverse outcome that may result from using EFT, Hypnosis or any alternative health care.

The Center for Inner Healing and Ted Robinson assume no liability for any reader or third party for any damages or injury which may result from utilizing anything contained within this book.

"Hypnosis is the most effective way of giving up smoking, according to the largest scientific comparison."
- New Scientist Magazine

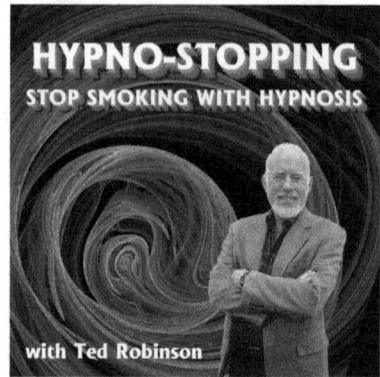

HYPNO-STOPPING
Stop Smoking with Hypnosis
$24.95 plus $4.99 S&H
Hypnosis is the best way to stop smoking. By adding EFT to the hypnosis process, you can also eliminate those old emotional urges that tempt you to smoke again.

Hypnosis and Emotional Freedom Technique, when used together, are the most powerful combination in use today to help you become a non-smoker for life.

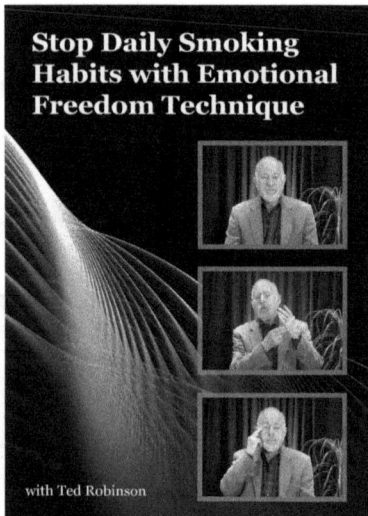

STOP DAILY SMOKING HABITS WITH EMOTIONAL FREEDOM TECHNIQUE
$29.95 plus $4.99 S&H
By adding Emotional Freedom Technique to the process, we can eliminate the potential for those old urges coming back and tempting you to smoke again. The two techniques, hypnosis and Emotional Freedom Technique, are absolutely the most effective means of ending your lifetime smoking habit and making you into a non-smoker for life.

Use this video to eliminate any and all habitual urges to smoke throughout the day that may hit you. We all know that we form habits like smoking while reading the paper, during the drive to work, at your coffee break and so on. This video will help you break those habits and once broken, they will not return. The videos are arranged to help you with your urges from the moment you get out of bed all the way to getting up in the middle of the night for that one last cigarette and everything in between. Let us help you become a non-smoker - FOR LIFE!

STOP EMOTIONAL URGES TO SMOKE WITH EFT
$29.95 plus $4.99 S&H
By adding Emotional Freedom Technique to the hypnosis process, you eliminate the potential for those old emotional urges to tempt you to smoke again. Hypnosis and Emotional Freedom Technique, when used together, will help you remain a non-smoker for life.

Stop Emotional Urges to Smoke with EFT
Emotional Freedom Technique

With
Ted Robinson

We know that in many situations, emotions arise that can trigger your urge to smoke. You can use this DVD to eliminate those emotional urges to smoke once and for all. The videos are arranged by specific emotions. Use the chapter menu to go directly to the video that addresses your emotional issue and tap along with it. It will help you remain a non-smoker - FOR LIFE!

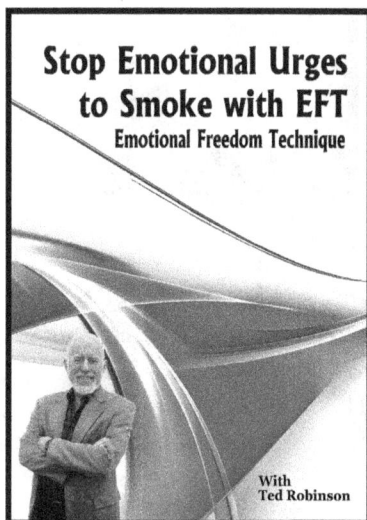

If you liked this book and want to learn more about our smoking cessation products, visit our website at innerhealingpress.com.

You may contact Ted Robinson by phone at (516) 248-5346 or by email at ted@tedrobinson.com

Other books by Theodore W. Robinson:

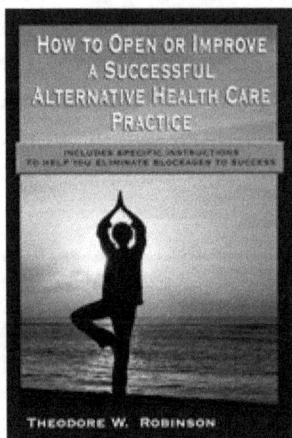

**HOW TO OPEN AND IMPROVE
A SUCCESSFUL ALTERNATIVE
HEALTH CARE PRACTICE**
$29.95 plus $4.99 S&H
This book will help you become the professional you can be in the burgeoning field of alternative health care. It contains marketing information, credit repair advice and a host of other things you will need to open your own practice or to improve an existing practice.

**108 WAYS TO MARKET
YOUR PRACTICE**
$24.95 plus $4.99 S&H
This book is a practical guide for success for holistic and alternative health care practitioners. It has a heavy emphasis on web related marketing techniques and unique ideas on how to jump start a new practice. There many additional topics including Unique Selling Propositions, how to overcome procrastination and eliminating resistance to change.

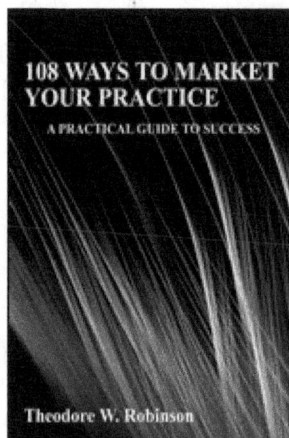

There is an entire appendix which teaches how to do Emotional Freedom Technique (EFT) and gives specific wording to achieve business success. This book will help everyone from the beginner to the seasoned practitioner with new ideas, new methods and unique approaches to achieve success.

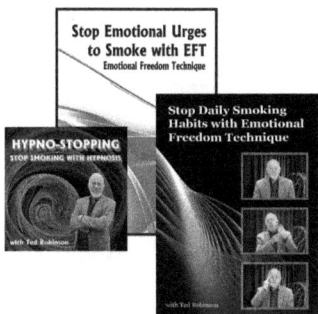

ORDER FORM

BUY THE SMOKING CESSATION PACKAGE (2 VIDEOS AND 1 CD) AND SAVE $25!!!
($70.07 plus $4.99 S&H)

Title	Qty.	Price w/ S&H	Total
☐ Hypno-Stopping Stop Smoking with Hypnosis	_____	x $29.94	_____
☐ Stop Daily Smoking Habits with Emotional Freedom Technique	_____	x $34.94	_____
☐ Stop Emotional Urges with EFT Emotional Freedom Technique	_____	x $34.94	_____
☐ **SAVE $25!!!** Smoking Cessation Package (includes the 2 DVDs and 1 CD above)	_____	x $75.06	_____
☐ How to Open and Improve a Successful Alternative Health Care Practice	_____	x $34.94	_____
☐ 108 Ways to Market Your Practice	_____	x $29.94	_____
		Total:	_____

Ship to:
Name: _____
Address: _____
_____

Send Check or Money Order only to:
Theodore W. Robinson
26 St. Paul's Place
Hempstead, NY 11550

www.ingramcontent.com/pod-product-compliance
Lightning Source LLC
Chambersburg PA
CBHW060854280326
41934CB00007B/1039